Guidebook on Helping Persons with Mental Retardation Mourn

Jeffrey Kauffman

Death, Value and Meaning Series
Series Editor: John D. Morgan

Baywood Publishing Company, Inc.
AMITYVILLE, NEW YORK

Baywood Publishing Company, Inc.
26 Austin Avenue
Amityville, NY 11701
(800) 638-7819
E-mail: baywood@baywood.com
Web site: baywood.com

Library of Congress Catalog Number: 2004054407
ISBN: 0-89503-300-3 (cloth)

Library of Congress Cataloging-in-Publication Data

Kauffman, Jeffrey.
    Guidebook on helping persons with mental retardation mourn / Jeffrey Kauffman.
       p. cm. -- (Death, value, and meaning series)
    Includes bibliographical references and index.
    ISBN 0-89503-300-3 (cloth)
    1. People with mental disabilities--Mental health. 2. People with mental
disabilities--Psychology. 3. People with mental disabilities--Counseling of. 4. Death. 5.
Grief. 6. Bereavement. I. Title. II. Series.

    RC451.4.M47K38 2004
    155.9'37'0874--dc22   2004054407

Contents

Preface

This book is primarily for: 1) mental retardation service providers, and for other persons who are concerned about the psychological and spiritual well-being of persons with mental retardation—families, advocates, and academics; and 2) grief counselors, therapists, and theorists. This book is also for psychotherapists who treat persons with mental retardation. I hope they will find the book useful in understanding the diverse expressions of grief in persons with mental retardation.

This text is intended to help lay a foundation for grief support services, to help establish standards of care, and to be an educational primer about the loss and mourning needs of persons with mental retardation. There is a need:

1. to recognize and conceptualize loss and mourning in persons with mental retardation;
2. to evolve practice standards and guidelines for agencies.

I hope that this book will contribute to the development of an awareness of the significance of loss in the life experience of persons with mental retardation. Experiencing loss is a very powerful vulnerability in their mental or psychological life, and is a basic element in psychological health.

The expressions of grief in persons with mental retardation also provides a window into the mourning process in a way that may deepen our understanding of grief and mourning in human beings, generally.

Acknowledgments

I want to thank the many people who have given me invaluable support and guidance in the course of my learning about the loss of mourning needs of persons with mental retardation. In 1988, while conducting a workshop on loss and mourning for PATH (People Acting to Help), a community mental health center in Philadelphia, staff from the agency's mental retardation division who had come to the workshop raised questions about the grief issues of a client whose mother had just died. In our discussion I realized that these experienced, perceptive, and caring staff persons were at a complete loss in knowing what to do to help this grieving client. After the workshop I learned that the literature on grief issues of persons with mental retardation was very scant. And, I came to see that mental retardation service providers had no conceptual frame of reference or practice guidelines for dealing with loss and grief issues, but did have an awareness of the need to develop and provide grief support services.

As I began to meet mental retardation program directors in the Philadelphia area, I was heartened at the welcome of many who were glad to collaborate with me in developing grief support services. I am grateful to the many administrators and staff who shared with me their knowledge and experience, and the many persons with mental retardation who have shared with me their grief and their selves.

Shortly after the training at PATH, I called the Philadelphia Office of Mental Retardation. Kathy Sykes, who was director of the office, assigned two staff to connect me up with agencies with whom I could explore the need for services, and begin to develop grief support services and models. Joe Bucci and his staff at TAIG, especially Murray Seligman, were generous in their support, and enabled me to begin to interview clients. Bonni Zedik of PDDC provided me with valuable help and opportunities to meet with workshop members at her agency. I am grateful to Alice Herzon of the Philadelphia Alliance of Mental Health Providers who helped me see needs and possibilities, and who introduced me to other agencies where I continued to meet clients who taught me about their loss and mourning needs. Jim Conroy's interest and repeated support has been crucial, and is deeply appreciated. Montgomery County (PA) Mental Retardation Administrator, Mariann Roach was very helpful in enabling me to provide services. Of the many agencies that have helped me in the development of these services, I especially want to thank Residential Support Systems of Ardmore, Pennsylvania, John Nicely, Director, and the exceptional team that works with him. I wish to express my appreciation for the opportunity to work with the concerned and dedicated staff of Indian Creek, and the many other agencies have given me the opportunity to learn from the staff and clients, including, The Whitelock Center of Devereux Foundation, PATH, Speaking for Ourselves, Elwyn, Delaware County Mental Retardation office, Barbar Associates, Philadelphia ARC and Delaware County (PA) ARC, Brian's House, Interact, Woodhaven Center, Community Interaction, The Salvation Army, Spin, Developmental Enterprises Corporation, Horizon House, Ken Crest, Mental Retardation Nurses Association of Philadelphia, Cerebral Palsy Association of Swarthmore, Pennsylvania, Community Options, Access Services, Networks for Training and Development. New Foundations, COMAR, JEVS, Lower Merion Vocational Center, and Step By Step. I also want to thank the many families who gave me the opportunity to work with and learn from them. And thanks to John Woestendiek and Angela Cato for talking with me about the story of Nicholas that appears in Chapter 3.

Thanks to attorney Dennis Mc Andrews for suggestions on the legal issues families need to be concerned with in preparation for the death of the primary caregiver.

I want to thank the Pennsylvania Department of Public Welfare, Developmental Disabilities Planning Council, who gave me a "small special projects grant," # 852731490, that ran from October 1, 1993 to September 30, 1994. This grant helped me provide some of these services. This book is the long overdue final phase of that project.

Special thanks to Hilda Kauffman, whose felicitous pen has revised and improved the language of this text and prepared it for publication. Her encouragement helped me to complete this book.

This book is a thank you note to all the agencies and staff persons, and especially the persons with mental retardation, from whom I have learned.

CHAPTER 1

Loss is At the Heart of Life: A General Introduction to Grief and the Practice of Helping Persons Who are Mourning

THE PERSON WHO GIVES GRIEF SUPPORT

Knowledge of the Grief of Others

There is much suffering in human life. The pain of death and of other losses, the grief experienced in diverse ways over the course of life, binds us together and divides us as human beings. *Caring for the losses of others* reaches across the divide between one human and another. Yet, is it really possible to know the pain of others? While our own death anxiety may close us off to the pain of others, and even to our own pain, concern for the grief of others is, no less, a basic part of our human identity; and our own moral or spiritual development may be based upon the maturation of our capacity to be receptive to and accepting of the pain of others. Our own grief anxiety, a possible impediment to compassion, then becomes the touchstone by which we become attuned to the grief of others. As a guidebook, the most basic concern of this little book is in *strengthening the grief support environment's ability to be responsive to the expressions of grief in persons with mental retardation.*

The grief counselor or therapist who approaches working with persons with mental retardation for the first time may feel like he or she is approaching a new territory, and confronting challenges that will require new knowledge and skills. This is only partially true.

Grief is grief, and once it is recognized how the person with mental retardation is *expressing* grief, and the grief counselor/therapist *recognizes* what the grief that is expressed *is saying*, then he or she will no longer be on unfamiliar ground. The greatest hurdle for the grief counselor/therapist is simply unfamiliarity with this client population, especially 1) the ways that persons with mental retardation express themselves and their grief, and 2) the social support structures in which the client lives. The grief counselor/therapist may, using this book as a guide, begin to familiarize him or herself with persons with mental retardation and their supportive environments, and may expect that competence will develop in the course of *learning from experience*. This guidebook will give the grief counselor/therapist a working perspective on and a basic understanding of how persons with mental retardation express grief and on their supportive living environments.

For families, advocates, and agencies the challenge is in being unfamiliar with grief, its expressions in persons with mental retardation, and how to think about the supports that may be developed to help facilitate the mourning process. This book may be used as a guide in beginning to understand grief in human beings, which includes themselves as well as persons with mental retardation, how persons with mental retardation express grief, and how to develop grief support. The recognition of expressions of grief and of the significance of grief support in the lives of persons with mental retardation, along with specific guidelines for program development spelled out here, set standards of care for agencies to strive toward.

While this guidebook aims to help persons who support grieving persons with mental retardation with *knowledge* about expressions of grief in persons with mental retardation, and with knowledge about the development of grief support services for persons with mental retardation—in a more basic sense, the book is intended to increase *awareness* of the psychological and spiritual grief language and vulnerabilities of persons with mental retardation. This awareness compels the development of norms for supporting the grief of persons with mental retardation.

The Caregivers Awareness of
His or Her Own Mortality

Openness to others and openness to oneself are really two aspects of the same openness to human mortality. This is because of the deep and intricate ways that the self's relationship with itself and the self's relationship with others are connected with regard to death and grief. One's own denials and dissociations of death anxiety in relation to oneself, may, in reaction to the grief of others, block our empathy or open it up. When one recognizes that one's reactions to the grief of others arouses one's own death anxiety, then one is in the position to learn from this awareness, and transform one's own grief from being an impediment to being the very touchstone of empathic support. Our own grief is always there in some way in our every encounter with the grief of others. It may be both an impediment and a means of empathic connection at the same time, but it is always there, and from the *way* that it is in the way there is something to learn.

Identifying with the grief of the other, such as a person with mental retardation, one may be threatened by the pain of one's own grief anxieties that one has not faced (or reckoned with well enough). Being aware of what is painful for oneself in the grief of others, including being aware of one's own denial, minimizing, rationalizing, and the desire to "fix" the pain of others (and oneself) and being gentle but firm with oneself about maintaining this awareness— helps to open up in oneself empathic receptive capacities.

Denial of identification with the grief of others may occur— 1) as anger at the bereaved for their disturbing grief behaviors, 2) as compulsive defenses that give one a sense of control by distancing oneself and pathologizing the grief behavior of the other, 3) in muted, numbed or basically indifferent reactions, or 4) in being overwhelmed by the grief of the other.

Denying the grief of others and turning a blind eye to oneself are two sides of the same anxiety. Becoming aware, here, really means *mourning*, which is a way a person opens inwardly to a core meaning of what it is to be human. Maybe all that we *know* about ourselves and others, and everything else we know, all knowing, is but compensation for failures of compassionate openness to the grief of others. And, maybe, our own most subjective pain and awareness of mortality have more to do with the grief of others than we have imagined.

As one begins and continues in helping others with grief, paying attention to one's own self, to one's own defenses against being aware of and receptive to the pain of others, helps us develop our sensitivity to the grief of others. For each of us, as we approach the work of supporting others in their grief and facilitating the mourning process, we approach a place which is spiritually and psychologically very powerful, both healing and dangerous. The caregiver should be prepared with self-awareness and an openness to the vulnerability of self and others and to the great spiritual and psychological wounds that occur in grief.

We know our own grief pain by experiencing a pain that comes up in oneself before one has words to say what it is. Sometimes, when we come to have words for our pain, we lose touch with the painfulness of it. Compassion calls one out of this forgetfulness of the very mortality that, in the first place, makes us human. It may be in some ways unsanctioned and unpleasant to allow oneself very much awareness of the grief of others. The norms of behavior in our culture do not give *real* social value to compassion, and, perhaps, this is inherent in that aspect of our nature that is often called *political*. Social norms of relating to others that are based in more unyielding forms of the denial of grief and death inform and are deeply rooted in each individual self. In a culture where empathy is deeply suspected of being a form of powerlessness, and as such is not subjectively trusted, the practice of compassionate care falters. Compassion is the *courage* to face the denial of grief and death in oneself. This compassion, or courage, is the basis of knowledge about grief, and knowledge based compassion is the basis of skill in providing grief support, counseling, or psychotherapy.

The Very Psychological Development of the Self is a Process of Mourning Losses

Over the course of a lifetime there are, for every person, many losses that happen. Every loss involves grief and a psychological process of responding to the grief that aims to repair the injury. This healing process may be called mourning. While birth is the first decisive loss experienced, a loss of being part of mother's body, loss of the womb, the loss that is our portal into being, is recapitulated throughout the process of becoming self. The separation-individuation process tells a story of becoming oneself (or, individuated) *through* a separation process. The negotiation of each step is a mourning process. The separation-individuation process is a process of becoming self through mourning a series of attachment losses, or separations.

The progression toward individuation and autonomy is a process of mourning/integrating a developmental sequence of losses. The core of the self, in this account, is a mourning process.

The *developmental norms* in this process are no different for persons with mental retardation than for others. But they may, for several reasons, be more complicated to negotiate for persons with mental retardation. These reasons have to do, on the one hand, with difficulties in one's experience of oneself in the world—doing things, communicating, relating to others, and getting one's needs met, and on the other hand, psychological processing interferences with mourning having to do, for example, with excesses of compulsivity and impulsivity.

For a person with mental retardation there are often loss experiences related to how he or she has experienced him or herself socially and subjectively over the course of growing up, and continuing into adulthood. Autonomy frustrations may contribute to an underlying grief in which there is vulnerability to narcissistic injury. Complications in the separation-individuation process of persons with mental retardation, and in how the person experiences him or herself in the process, contribute to vulnerabilities in the mourning process.

Throughout life, unto the final loss, the loss of life (death), loss and responses to loss, inscribed in the self, shape our human identity. Along with this process of becoming a self through the development of the ability to mourn, there are many losses that leave their mark on a person.

In the impact of loss, and the process of mourning loss becomes saturated with meaning around which the identity of the self develops. What happens in the mourning process is the heart of a person's life; in the sense in which loss and mourning shapes identity, self-valuation, and other basic assumptions about oneself and the world, and fosters cohesion of the self, mourning is at the heart of individual human life.

Mourning is a vital aspect of the psychological, spiritual, and moral well-being of the whole person, both in one's relationship with oneself (as in one's self-concept), and in one's relationship with the world (as in social adjustment). Grief is not isolated to a narrow band of the person's life; when someone is grieving, their most human vulnerabilities may be at stake, 1) the confidence of attachment to others and to oneself, 2) belief in the secure continuity of oneself, and 3) a sense of self-worth.

In this book we look at the lives of persons with mental retardation through a lens that focuses in on experiences of loss at the heart of psychological existence and health.

SUPPORTING THE MOURNING PROCESS
OF OTHERS

Recognizing Grief and Facilitating the Mourning Process

When a loss is experienced—whether the loss is the death of a loved one, a relationship otherwise broken, a change in one's life, a disappointment, or a loss of self, such as an injury to one's self-concept or self-worth—grief is triggered. Grief is the psychological reaction to an experience of loss; it is a disturbance that affects a person's relationship with himself or herself and with the social environment. Grief is a disruption of the orderliness and predictability of one's world. It is a longing, an emptiness and abandonment, a broken attachment. It is the utter helplessness to get back what is lost. It is the pain of losing (some part of) oneself. It is a broken connection. It is the humiliation of being subjected to these losses. It is a terrible anxiety that is aroused that may threaten ones sense of self and security, undermine one's sense of meaningfulness, hope, and existence.

Whenever grief is experienced the grief-stricken person needs to *process the loss* and the disruptive psychological occurrences associated with the injury, which have both affective and cognitive components. Grief occurs in the lives of persons with mental retardation no differently than in persons without mental retardation, though aspects of the *expression* of grief, of the subjective processing of grief, and typical patterns of complicated mourning may differ. While grief is grief in human beings, there are some special concerns that we are faced with in recognizing and understanding the grief of persons with mental retardation, and in supporting their mourning process.

There had been a time when it was widely believed that persons with mental retardation did not experience grief. This was a particularly de-humanizing presumption. Furthermore, this probably means that it was a fact of existence for some persons with mental retardation that grief occurred inwardly, but was as confusing and incoherent to the self of the person with mental retardation as it was unrecognized and unsanctioned by the social environment.

The connection between social recognition and psychological experience of self, on the one hand, and grief, on the other, is, that the psychological self is prone to experience itself and its grief *in accordance with implicit and explicit social expectations*. In other words, a significant aspect of the self's experience of itself is experiencing itself in the eyes of others. When grief is not socially recognized, the reality and very existence of grief is prone to be excluded from consciousness, or, at least unsupported and undermined, *while the pain of the loss persists, disconnected from the self's awareness;* and when grief is excluded from consciousness, it is prone to become a "psychological dysfunction." A behavior may be recognized as a problem without recognizing that it is expressing grief. This may be so, e.g., with aggressive behaviors, self-hurting behaviors, relationship difficulties, somatic complaints, social withdrawal, depression, etc. A behavior may be seen to be characteristic of an individual, without recognizing the origin of the pattern of behavior in a *loss* experience.

In order to help people with their mourning process, we need to recognize grief when we see it. When a loss is not evident, that is, when there is no link recognized between the loss event and the grief behavior, the behavior is seen to be a behavioral or mental health problem. A behavior may be recognized as a problem without recognizing that it is expressing grief, typically aggressive behaviors, increased frustration, increased compulsivity, self-hurting behaviors, relationship difficulties, somatic complaints, and even social withdrawal.

Ken Doka (1989, 2002) introduced the term "disenfranchised grief" for grief that is not socially recognized, and so is unsanctioned. Persons with mental retardation may be vulnerable to not recognizing their own grief *as grief*. If, for example, the environment mistakes an aggressive expression of grief to be an expression of selfishness or manipulation ("he is just being angry because he wants to get his way"), or takes grief to be a medication problem or some behavioral or psychiatric disorder, then the person's grief is *disenfranchised*. As a consequence the person is subject to the injury of being invisible in a most vulnerable time of need for social support. When grief is not recognized, the person is especially prone to damage to the sense of self and to problem behaviors.

Grief that has no social context, or an inadequate social context in which to be experienced is at increased risk of becoming depression, aggression, withdrawal, or other symptoms, no longer recognized as expressions of grief. This grief may lodge in the self, and become a part of the self, in the sense of becoming a personality trait. Sometimes when a loss is experienced, there is a regression along the self's most vulnerable fault lines. Inwardly, disenfranchised grief puts one at odds with oneself in having experienced the *impact* of loss without the social and cultural supports that allow one to grieve. The communities in which a person with mental retardation lives are the social environments *in which he experiences himself;* so, grief support needs to begin with *recognition of grief by the community in which the person lives.* Simply providing an adequate social context for the person to experience his grief is the most basic sense of facilitating the mourning process. This book gives guidelines and recommendations for how to provide this *recognition.* Recognition is the most basic and far-reaching form of support and way of facilitating the mourning process.

As best as I have been able to tell, there was no literature, and little practice of recognizing the grief of persons with mental retardation before the mid-1970s. Some initial literature on death and persons with mental retardation, while, for example, recognizing the need for the person to attend a funeral, was mainly concerned with teaching "appropriate" behavior for the event. As the grief of persons with mental retardation was first acknowledged, there was concern with justifying the fact that persons with mental retardation actually grieved. Today it is widely recognized that persons with mental retardation grieve, and needing to justify the fact of grief would betray a failure to recognize the humanity of persons with mental retardation.

With an evolution of awareness and knowledge about the emotional life of persons with mental retardation, significantly increased respect for their dignity, and evolving standards of care, *plus* advances in recognizing the grief needs of persons with mental retardation that have occurred in an emergent literature standards of grief support have begun to develop. Support environments often 1) aim to be thoughtful and sensitive about how a person is informed about a death, 2) provide ritual opportunities for recognition of a loss, 3) provide other grief processing opportunities, 4) provide interpersonal support, and 5) refer for grief counseling or therapy when more complicated grief reactions occur, or routinely do so when a loss happens (which is a less common practice, but a good one). There is a caring recognition of the existence of grief, and a recognition that there is more that needs to be learned about grief support. This guidebook is the report of a grief therapist who has worked with families, agencies, and persons with mental retardation, and has tried to understand the grief needs that presented themselves. This is written with the hope that it will contribute to the continued development of *standards of grief care* for mental retardation service providers and the continued development of our understanding of the expressive language of grief and the grief needs of persons with mental retardation.

Recognizing Grief is the Basic Supportive Response to Grief

The very act of recognizing grief goes a long way in facilitating the mourning process. When we talk here about recognizing grief the term "recognize" is meant in two ways. To recognize grief means, on the one hand, simply to be aware of it. But, it also means to socially express the recognition, to respond to a grieving person in ways that recognizes his or her grief. We must be aware of the person's grief before we can socially recognize it. It is, however, the second sense of *recognition* that helps specifically to facilitate the mourning process. There are many ways we may express recognition of grief. We express recognition, for example, by:

1. interpersonally acknowledging grief,
2. establishing situations in which the grieving person may acknowledge grief,
3. integrating a recognition of the mourning needs of persons with mental retardation into program support design,
4. understanding and responding to the behavioral language of grief, and
5. understanding the ways that grief reactions may be protracted, detached from the event of the loss, and behaviorally expressed over many, many years, even until death.

Sometimes the supportive environment initiates recognition of a loss, and supports the person's involvement in rituals, or provides other activities to memorialize a loss. Other times, the supportive environment is responsive to the grieving person's expressions of grief. An agency may also establish conditions in which grief is recognized and supported by agency procedures and protocols, such as doing a loss assessment during the admission process, providing staff training in loss and grief, or in any other way that establishes agency recognition of grief. These topics will be discussed in Chapter 6, "Program Development." For the grief counselor and therapist (and for others in the supportive environment as well) recognition of the loss is defined by the special interactive nature of the relationship, in which recognition specifically occurs in the empathic attunement to the person and to his/her expressions of grief.

Grief is a Disturbance

Grief is a disturbance. This may seem self-evident. But, there is a normal human tendency to dispel, shun, defend against, pathologize, and ignore the very disturbing nature of grief as much as possible. We should never underestimate the power of the urge to deny grief. Humans have a limited capacity for tolerating grief, and only the force of pain, and inward disturbances, keeps grief present.

The distinction between normal grief and grief that is not normal (which used to be called pathological grief, and is now usually called complicated grief) is often a great concern for grief experts, and for persons facing grief in their personal lives. Mourning is, itself, a normative concept, and the act of mourning instantiates norms. But, perhaps, this distinction no less reflects our anxiety about having or knowing the acceptable boundaries for the disturbing and disruptive forces of grief. And, if we can establish these boundaries, that is, make the distinction between normal and not normal, and if we are confident about what is over the line, not normal and to be excluded from our self-permitted range of experience, then anxiety may be reduced.

A practical reason for the environment that supports persons with mental retardation to make the distinction between normal and not normal grief may be to know when a referral to a grief counselor or therapist is indicated. But, there is no need to identify a grief reaction as not normal in order to refer for an evaluation by a grief specialist. Referral for grief evaluation by a grief counselor/ therapist, or grief evaluation by knowledgeable agency staff, may be a rule of thumb, a part of the process of recognizing the loss. Treatment may, then, be indicated when, 1) the person's language of grief, as we shall see in subsequent chapters, expresses that they are experiencing a level of distress that is overwhelming coping capacities, or 2) an affective intensity of grief is expressed that concerns others who know the person, or 3) there are significant behavioral changes.

In any case, because of the disturbance and pain of the experience of loss, loss is defended against in various ways, but it is always defended against. The very extendedness of grief over time, its temporality, and the psychodynamics, which are activated in grief, involve an interaction of grief and the denial of grief. The process usually called mourning is set in motion by the tension between the impact of the loss, including the meaning of the loss, and the denial or dissociation of the loss. When we approach the disturbance incited by loss we are guided by cognizance of the power of grief disturbances and of the meaningfulness of barriers erected in the face of these disturbances.

While we are concerned here with the grieving individual's experiences of the disturbances of grief, the supportive environment also grieves, and a very similar process of interaction between experiencing a loss and defending against it occurs in the supportive environments of family, staff, advocates, grief professional, and the community at large. Social environments of persons with mental retardation react to the grief of a grieving person with a process, usually in the background behind professional roles and identities and tasks with a process of being impacted and defending against the impact and meaning of the experience. The grief reactions of the supportive environment that are occurring in reaction to the grief of the person who is being supported, are a key part of the *supportiveness* of the supportive environment.

Any social environment has a strong defensive motive in face of the grief disturbance of other persons within the environment. The defensive motive in the face of grief is there in each person in face of the otherness of the death of others, as well as the otherness of his own death. The environment defends in many ways against the grief of any individual person within the environment.

For helpers, denial of grief disturbances and of the meanings of these disturbances in the experience of the person helped, may mask itself as an intention to repair the damage and make the hurt go away. The supportive aim is not to fix the hurt, but to facilitate the mourning process: to recognize or acknowledge the loss and *support the expression of grief*.

Perhaps not every loss inflicts a significantly disturbing grief reaction. If a situation occurs in which there is a loss, but for the person it is not eventful, or does not appear to impact the person as a loss, then opportunities to acknowledge the loss should still be provided, but if there is no *experienced* loss for the person, there is no loss to be mourned. For example, if a parent dies and the person does not react, the supportive environment should still provide opportunities for the person to mourn, but, the death may not be a loss for that person, and the absence of grief does not mean it is missing, only being inhibited.

However, sometimes defenses against the loss shut down a grief reaction, so that it may appear there is no grief, but the impact of the loss takes its toll, and expressions of grief occur later, and in ways that may not, without a careful evaluation, appear to have any connection to the loss. Losses may not register consciously or be exhibited in order to shape a person's sense of identity, one's experience of oneself and others in the world, or how one loves. Losses that slip in under the radar screen, and never register consciously, may still be psychologically consequential, and the person's responses to the loss should, in this instance, still be noted in an ongoing psychosocial history that is especially concerned with losses. This account of losses by the community may turn out to be valuable over time.

Recognize the Diverse Kinds of Loss Experience that Occur in the Lives of Persons with Mental Retardation

Life is full of change and loss. For all the willfulness one may exercise to maintain the constancy of one's self and one's world, changes take place. This tension between constancy and change is there, no doubt, from the instant of birth, when the first change happens, throughout the time between birth and death, the final change. Every change is a loss of the *constancy* of the self and the world. The adaptive ability of a person is the ability to negotiate change, or the loss of constancy. The adaptive response seeks to re-establish a sense of the constancy of experience. Constancy and the disruption of constancy organize the experience of the self over time, so that compulsive trends develop over time in response to changes that threaten to overwhelm adaptive responses. Mourning involves: 1) reckoning with the painful disturbance of the loss, and 2) adaptive re-organization of experience of oneself and the world that has been disrupted.

This perspective on the mourning process, which is a general theory of the psychology of mourning, has particular meaning in understanding the grief and mourning of persons with mental retardation, among whom there is a marked tendency toward increased levels of compulsivity in reaction to change and loss.

There are many types of loss and change in the lives of persons with mental retardation. Here is a list of some common types of change and loss in the lives of persons with mental retardation:

1. loss of constancy, routine, familiarity, predictability, etc. This is also called "loss of the assumptive world" (Kauffman, 2002a).

2. loss of familiar place, such as change in workplace, or in residence.

3. death, especially, the death of a family member, friend, or staff person.

4. broken relationships other than due to death, such as family members who have withdrawn, staff turnover and transfer losses, broken peer relationships. Broken relationships from family members who have abandoned them and from staff turnover is a significant source of unrecognized grief among persons with mental retardation. Relationships may also be broken without the other person actually going away, due to conflict and rejection.

5. illnesses of self and others. Illness may arouse anxiety based on (a) physical changes in the other person or oneself, (b) death anxiety, (c) if the relationship to the sick person involves dependency or deep attachment, a loss of care or of a secure bond, and (d) memories of past experiences of illness.

6. loss-of-self or narcissistic anxiety. Loss of self refers to damage to the self-concept, self-worth, self-confidence, sense of competence, sense of belonging, or wounds to other aspects of a person's experience of him or herself. It may be caused or increased by (a) experiences of abandonment and disconnect, (b) experiences of social devaluation, (c) experiences of not being able, (d) experiences of frustration about limits of autonomy, (e) experiences of psychological helplessness, and (f) feelings of shame or humiliation in these experiences.

Injuries to the sense of self that occur while a person is growing up and becoming him or herself, including developing a sense identity, are prone to be an acutely present force in reaction to losses and narcissistic injuries throughout life.

7. the person with mental retardation may internalize their parents' losses and frustrations. Internalized fragments of unresolved

parental grief may become a part of one's sense of identity, passed on in the ways that the person experiences himself to be wounded in interpersonal interactions with the parent. Subsequent losses tend to wound in already established vulnerable places. So, it would be no surprise to discover that patterns of psychological woundedness that occur throughout a person's life, originate in negative experiences of oneself that occur in the relationship with parents. These injuries are a psychological undertow that affect the mourning process in all persons, and notably so, among person with mental retardation.

8. psychosocial losses, such as loss of a job.

9. losses with traumatic features. Experiences that violate the self, such as abuse, neglect, violence, rejection, abandonment, overwhelming guilt or shame, or any changes that totally overwhelm the ego's adaptive ability—set off a traumatic stress anxiety (Rando, 2000). There may be a particular vulnerability among persons with mental retardation for narcissistic injuries in grief to have traumatic features.

REFERENCES

Doka, K. (Ed). (1989). *Disenfranchised grief.* Lexington: Lexington Books/ D.C. Heath.

Doka, K. (Ed.) (2002). *Disenfranchised grief: New directions, challenges and strategies for practice.* Champaign: Research Press.

Kauffman, J. (2002). The psychology of disenfranchised grief. In K. Doka (Ed.), *Disenfranchised grief: New directions, challenges and strategies for practice.* Champaign: Research Press.

Kauffman, J. (Ed.) (2002a). *Loss of the assumptive world.* New York: Brunner-Routledge.

Rando, T. (2000). On the experience of traumatic stress in anticipatory and postdeath mourning. In T. Rando (Ed.), *Clinical dimensions of anticipatory mourning.* Champaign: Research Press.

CHAPTER 2

Guidelines for Supporting and Facilitating the Mourning Process

THE AIM OF THE SUPPORTIVE ENVIRONMENT IS TO FACILITATE THE MOURNING PROCESS

When a person is grieving the most basic task of the supportive environment is simply to provide opportunities for the person to safely experience his or her grief. Creating social and interpersonal environments, or creating clinical grief processing environments, where a person's grief is *recognized* and meaningfully respected as a vulnerability—facilitates the mourning process. Supporting a person in their grief, in very a basic sense, simply means to recognize, and to validate in a way that *supports the person's experience of their loss*, and, that supports the person's experience of *themselves* in grieving.

Grief support is both a knowledge-based skill, *and* a compassionate awareness of the grief that is experienced. This guidebook aims to provide the reader with the basic knowledge that will help him or her to become skillful at providing grief support. Skill is the ability to use knowledge about grief to effectively help facilitate the mourning process. But, there is another dimension beyond, or in addition to knowledge and skill, and that is compassionate awareness of the grief of the person with mental retardation. Awareness of grief is inherently compassionate, because simple and genuine awareness involves being touched by the other person's grief, and this compels one to either deny what one is touched by, or to respond with compassion. And to deny is to foreclose awareness. Being touched by another's grief, to the extent that awareness does not succumb to denial and inner deadness, calls us to recognize the other's pain, and to support the person in his grief; and doing so, humanizes us.

In persons with mental retardation there is the full range of human responses to death and other loss. Though the expressive language of grief among persons with mental retardation may, as we shall see, differ from the general population, the pain of grief, the meaningfulness of loss, the need for social support are common experiences of all human beings. Every grief response is taken to be a meaningful expression of grief, though it is not always evident what the meaning is. The supportive job is, in the first place: 1) to recognize what the grief language is saying, and 2) to decide how to supportively respond.

WHEN A DEATH HAPPENS:
GENERAL GUIDELINES

The four most important ingredients for supporting persons with mental retardation when a death happens are:

1. provide information and support the processing of information;
2. enable maximum involvement in the social environment surrounding the death;
3. do relationship work in the supportive relationship in which the aim is maximizing a sense of security, nurturing interpersonal reconciliation, nurturing opportunities for meaningful connectedness; and
4. maximize opportunities for self-expression.

When a death happens the need for *information*, connection to the social context of the death, cognitive and affective *self-expression*, and *relationship security* guide the intervention plan. Encourage maximum involvement in social contexts that recognize and give experiences of security and meaning to the loss, and that support safe passage through the sometime turbulent, sad, scary, and confusing experiences of grief.

When a death is anticipated, then the primary supportive task is to support *present* anxiety, grief related to *present* stressors, practical and emotional life complication due to the illness or changes in the appearance of the sick person, and changes in routines or other aspects of experience in which the familiar and expected is disrupted.

DOES A PERSON WITH MENTAL RETARDATION UNDERSTAND DEATH?

Thanatologists have approached the question of what it means to understand death by identifying a few concepts that are regarded as defining death; and, if a person grasps these concepts, it is said that they understand the concept of death. Two key concepts that define a persons understanding of death are called *irreversibility* and *non-functionality*. Irreversibility, which simply means that the deceased does not return, or that a person understands that dead means not coming back to life, seems to me to be commonly grasped by persons with mental retardation with whom I have communicated, with, generally, the same consistency of thought as persons without mental retardation. The concept of non-functionality, which means, and would more accurately and simply be called *not moving*, that is, not capable of moving oneself, is, I have found also to be commonly understood by persons with mental retardation.

In the case examples that follow there are instances in which behavior suggested that the concept of death was not understood, but in each case it turned out to have been me who didn't understand what the behavior was saying, and the person did indeed understand "the concept of death" with grasp similar to the grasp by persons who do not have mental retardation. All the grieving persons with moderate and mild mental retardation with whom I have worked grasp, in their lived experience of loss, the concept of irreversibility, and the firmness of this grasp does not appear to be less than that of other humans.

In the case of Chad cited in Chapter 4, we meet a man who talked about visiting his deceased aunt; he talked in a way that led his support staff and myself to believe that he did not grasp that she was gone. But, in fact his saying he wanted to visit his aunt did not indicate that he didn't know she was dead and was not coming back; he was, rather, expressing how he *missed* his family and how much he *wished* to visit his aunt's home. And, even though he may have had some confusion about her *really* and unequivocally being gone, he clearly grasped the concept of the irreversibility of death. While sometimes the grasp is equivocal in persons with mental retardation as it is with other human beings, the expression of these equivocations may be more candidly and concretely expressed.

It is sometimes very hard to discriminate between "not grasping irreversibility," on the one hand, and "denial" on the other—especially when the denial is expressed in behavior that assumes the deceased to be still alive, and so gives the impression that one has not understood that the person is, actually, dead. In the course of normal mourning recognition and denial of loss alternate; the normal process of integrating a loss involves the repeated occurrence of a state of mind in which a person may be gone, *but they are not really gone.* There may be a clear recognition that the person is gone, but a lot of mental equivocation about this. In persons with mental retardation, at least in mild and moderate mental retardation, it is typically no different, except, as we shall see, the language in which the equivocation is expressed is different.

One more thought about the concept of irreversibility: without a grasp, on some level, of irreversibility, the mourning process would not be a reckoning with the ultimate loss that, at the core of our psychological being, defines who we are as human beings—but, rather, with a loss in which there is no compelling need for a *decisive resignation* that the person is really gone, and not coming back; and so, there would be nothing to *compel* mourning, and it would not occur. It seems to me that recognition of the irreversibility of death is always, for all human beings, including persons with mental retardation, equivocal, and the mourning process is likewise, a kind of equivocation, in which acceptance that death is irreversible is never final.

It is a vain, though socially accepted self-deception and prevarication that persons without mental retardation grasp the concept of death, as, for example, expressed by the concept of irreversibility, with less ambiguity than persons with mental retardation.

BREAKING THE NEWS OF A DEATH

When a death occurs family or staff may be faced with the responsibility of breaking the news. Both telling and hearing are very tender and difficult experiences. The burden carried by the person who tells is his awareness of the vulnerability of the other that occurs upon hearing this news. The approach to breaking the news is to hold sacred the wound that the news of death may inflict. The person giving the news may express and carry himself or herself in a concerned, respectful, gentle way and speak directly, simply, and, sometimes, haltingly. The stance and manner of approach in breaking the news is a primary language by which a death is announced, even before the words are spoken. Learning of the death of a loved one is a moment when shock may overwhelm the ego, and a process is set in motion in which the ego integrates what is denied or dissociated in the moment of shock. So, the moment of hearing the news may have an impact that reoccurs during the mourning process.

Who should break the news? Someone who knows the person and who has an emotional connection should break the news. Ideally, the person who breaks the news is someone connected to the deceased and to the bereaved, someone who shares the grief and who is part of the social fabric in which the deceased and the bereaved are connected.

Experts in the field of death and dying have recommended that it is good to use the words *death* and *dead,* rather than euphemisms, and I think that word *death* does convey the "reality of death," or, at least, does not wink at death and support denial. A euphemism in breaking the news denies death, disenfranchises the griever. And for this reason straight, honest and simple language, expressed in a most unintrusive way (for the news is itself a very great intrusion), may help facilitate a mourning process. The *directness* of the words conveys the reality of death and gives permission to experience and express the pain of the loss. Grief support is *giving permission,* and straightforwardness in speaking of death is a way of giving permission to grieve. In breaking the news of a death one conveys information *and* gives permission to grieve. The way the news is broken to the bereaved conveys a message about societal expectations; breaking the news of a death functions as a social act of sanctioning the person as a griever.

We may with good sense expect that the bereaved will be devastated by the news. Initial reactions, however, vary greatly. Some persons may have a mild reaction; others may have little or no reaction. When the news of a death arrives, the anxiety that is aroused is likely to require significant defenses in order for the self to absorb and survive the blow. The reality of the news may be blocked out so that there is impact, but awareness has been split off, dissociated, until the ego can allow itself. The loss may sometimes not even *register*. It may take the experienced absence of the deceased person or a ritual acknowledgement for the person to begin to realize the loss. So recognizing and "taking in" the loss and reactions to the loss usually occurs over a very extended period of time. Breaking the news is the beginning of a process of mourning and, perhaps, living with the loss.

When there is a death of a resident or staff person, in which a group of clients are affected, the news should, when possible, be broken to the group of affected persons together. Group processing time is provided immediately after the announcement. Follow-up group meetings to further share feelings and support, and to process the loss, are also indicated.

BEGIN WITH AN ASSESSMENT

The grief support process begins with an assessment of the person's grief and aims to develop a plan to support the person in his or her grief and facilitate the mourning process. Assessing means figuring out what is going on, what the loss means, how the person is grieving, and vulnerabilities that may be pertinent to the person's experience of the loss. In some situations, such as grief counseling/ therapy or in agencies aiming to support persons expressing complicated grief, it means gathering all relevant information that may be affecting the person's experience of grief. In other instances, such as an agency supporting a person presenting uncomplicated grief, information gathering may be limited to the specific circumstances of and reactions to loss.

At the beginning of every helping relationship, and continuing over time, an assessment is conducted. This process also communicates to the grieving person a concern with their grief, and draws together and brings into view, hopefully, for both the griever and the helper, the scattered and confusing pain of grief. The process of assessing loss may help to define the person's experience of the loss.

Assessment is an act of gathering information, which also *engages* the mourning process. The information gathering aims to understand the person's *experience* of loss. Information is gathered for the purpose of composing a picture of what the griever is experiencing and the psychological and spiritual meaning of their pain, and to engage the griever, so far as possible, in the process of calling to attention and symbolizing the loss, in whatever way that may happen, even simply by indicating and identifying the loss or by being interested in and concerned about the loss. The assessment develops a story of the persons experience of grief, and includes, 1) an account of the factors that are affecting their grief, 2) how this grief is expressed, and 3) what the loss means.

Loss assessments should be done by agencies, especially residential agencies, but other agencies, as well, as a part of a broader assessment done in the course of the admissions process. Knowing the loss issues related to the placement or other changes concurrent with admission, and loss issues prior to current situation, are a basic part of the admission process. Losses are central to a psychosocial assessment, and provide important information about emotional vulnerabilities, as well as the process of adjusting to the new environment the person is entering. These and related concerns about initial agency loss assessments will be discussed below in the chapter on program development.

Here, we are mainly concerned with the assessment that is conducted in response to a person's experiencing a specific loss. The loss may be a death, a broken relationship (such as staff turnover, or the withdrawal of a family member), or any significant life change or disappointment. Death is a special case of a change that needs to be adapted to, and may be thought of as the root anxiety, that is, that any change means, psychologically, that permanence is illusory, and order and security are uncertain. Grief may be understood as the disturbance that occurs in reaction to change.

Changes in the behavior of the person who has experienced a loss are specific indicators of *grief distress,* and may also give an indication of adaptive and defensive measures deployed to cope, and of what adaptive pathways are needed and possible. *Changes in expressive-behavioral language subsequent to a loss focus the process of evaluation and intervention planning.* Behavioral expressions of grief, such as increased compulsivity, aggression, or withdrawal guide our thinking as we try to understand the griever's experience of the loss, as we gather information about possible past influences on the present experience, and as we develop and implement a support plan.

While important aspects of the assessment process are conducted in interviews with staff and family, the grieving person should be party to this process to the maximum degree possible. Generally, the person is interviewed both with others and alone. Family or support staff inclusion in grief counseling/therapy sessions is discussed later in this chapter in the section called "The collaborative relationship between grief counselor/therapist and agency or family." The assessment process continues over the course of the helping relationship, as grief behaviors and feelings continue to occur, and as the helping relationship unfolds and evolves.

An essential part of the assessment process, a part in which the mourning process is particularly facilitated is helping the person to self-evaluate, to identify for him or herself the meaning of the behavior, the presence of grief, the thoughts and feelings associated with this, his or her wishes and needs, etc. Facilitating self-evaluation is an integral part of supporting the mourning process, and occurs not just at the outset, but throughout the time that the person is grieving, however long that may be.

Past loss experiences should be evaluated for their bearing upon present grief. Old losses may influence how present losses are experienced. Broken relationships, including losses from death, major disappointments, and narcissistic injuries should be considered. While it occurs with all persons, persons with mental retardation are especially prone to re-experience aspects of past grief in reaction to present losses. This tendency may be related to a vulnerability to traumatic stress anxiety or to a proclivity for compulsivity, which preserves the currency of long past grief experiences. In any case, the wounds of past losses are a regressive undertow when a new loss occurs. So, knowing the history of losses may, in some cases, provide very useful information for understanding the experience and meaning of the present loss that is being evaluated.

While the psychological drama experienced in a loss is triggered by diverse factors, I want to note three particular areas of concern: (1) the *relationship* with the deceased (or the person with whom a relationship has been broken), (2) *circumstances related to the event* of death or the otherwise broken relationship, and (3) injuries to the sense of self, or *narcissistic injuries* that are experienced in the loss, including the wounds of broken attachments.

(1) Assess Relationship with the Deceased

We want to try to understand what the broken relationship meant, and what the attachment experience was. The broken attachment bond may trigger separation anxiety and abandonment anxiety, which are often at the heart of grief; separation and abandonment anxieties are experienced in diverse aspects of grief, such as insecurity, loneliness, self-blame, and feelings of devaluation. Conflicts, frustrations, and hurt and angry feelings that have existed in the relationship may be persistent and complicated in mourning the loss of the relationship. Frustrations in the relation may occur in grief as the psychological meaning of the loss. For example, when Candace's mother died the abandonment she felt was an intensification of abandonment and rage she'd felt over the history of the relationship. In another case, Henry's father died and the guilt and anger that overcame him was the same guilt and anger he'd felt since early childhood in his relationship with his father. We want to understand the disturbing aspects of the relationship to look for how it may be playing out in the grief over the loss.

(2) Assess Circumstances Related to the Death or Loss

Carefully review the circumstances around the ending of the relationship, with particular attention to how the person experienced the end of the relationship. How did the ending happen, and what did it mean for the person? How was the person involved or left out? Was there adequate opportunity for goodbyes to be said, and what did this mean for the person? What circumstances of the death or loss have emotional significance for the person? What changes in the person's life occurred as a consequence of loss? What social supports have there been, and, more importantly what is the person's perception of his social support?

(3) Assess Injuries to the Sense of Self

Persons with mental retardation appear to be particularly vulnerable to injuries to their sense of self, damage to the self-concept, an insult to the sense of self-worth, and feelings of abandonment— as complicating factors in grief. Aggression in the grief reaction may be due to a variety of factors, but is often an expression of the narcissistic injury and frustration of being abandoned. Impulsive aggressions in persons with mental retardation may be expressions of feeling a loss to be an assault that violates and annihilates oneself.

ACCEPTANCE, AFFIRMATION, AND
VALIDATION OF GRIEF

We should not underestimate, and we cannot overestimate, the simple power of acceptance, affirmation, and validation. It is the key to supporting grief. The pain of grief, the burden carried, even the psychological complications that may emerge in grief, are eased, and the mourning process facilitated, by the power of acceptance, affirmation, and validation. A person is pained and hurt by grief in such a way that invalidates personhood. Unaccepted, disavowed or ignored, and invalidated grief undermines belief in oneself, the safety and value of one's existence. To accept, affirm, and validate provides a sanctuary for grief disturbances.

Accepting and validating are the basic principles of the helping relationship that are paramount in supporting the grieving process. In recognizing a loss, the support process aims to give acceptance, affirmation, and validation to the grief injured self, such as undermining one's self-concept. Feeling abandoned, for example, exposes the grieving person to shame about ones own value and existence. Acceptance, affirmation, and validation help protect against and heal these diverse narcissistic vulnerabilities.

SYMBOLIZATION

An important aspect of the mourning process is symbolization. By symbolizing I mean the process of transforming the disturbing subjectivity aroused by death, loss, and trauma, into the reality of symbolic representations. Mourning is a process of creating symbolic meanings that provide cover and safety in face of anxiety about the raw, overwhelming reality of death. Mourning transforms death by making symbolic sense, or meaning or cognitive coherence, in the face of the senseless violence and unpredictability of death, and anxieties that are related to this, such as annihilation, helplessness, and abandonment anxiety—which are at the core of grief. The process of mourning draws together the underlying loss anxieties into a symbolic reality that integrates the loss, while at the same time aspects of loss and grief continue to exist outside the symbolic reality constructed through mourning.

I am making special note of the psychological process of symbolization in grief, because the basic symbolizing function of mourning, and its limitations, are not well enough understood; I want to draw attention to symbolization especially, with the hope of dispelling the belief that persons with mental retardation cannot symbolically represent death and loss. Among *all* persons we find cultural symbolic and narratives that give a sense of hope, security, and meaning, and that help bind affective and cognitive disturbances that occur in grief, and shape the identity of the self.

The basic supportive process of recognizing the loss and validating the griever facilitates the symbolization of grief, and the relationship with another person or a supportive community provides experiences in which the loss is symbolized. In addition to providing a safe, supportive world in which the person may live, the symbolization process may be facilitated in such particular practices as:

1. helping the person put thoughts and feelings into *words*;
2. helping the person find *expressive language* to symbolize grief. This may be done by creating rituals or other memorialization events, activities and behaviors, such as discussed in the next section "Facilitate active and maximum participation in social experience of the loss and facilitate activities for the person to experience the loss," in the second part called "Doing things."
3. recognizing and validating the symbolization expressed behaviorally by the person.
4. making *links* between (a) affects and behaviors that express grief and (b) the loss.
5. help the person find answers for questions raised by loss, such as, "did she die because I was a bad person?" (This is abandonment anxiety with a narcissistic regression to self-referential grief thoughts, and an attempt to bind the abandonment anxiety by guilt.) Or, in the case of a man who sits at the door of his residence with his suitcase packed, waiting for his deceased father, he is asking a question about his father's absence.

The grief counselor or therapist and the broad supportive environment help the grieving person make sense out of the pain and senselessness of death by supporting the mourning process in the diverse ways discussed in this guidebook.

FACILITATE ACTIVE AND MAXIMUM PARTICIPATION IN SOCIAL EXPERIENCE OF THE LOSS AND FACILITATE ACTIVITIES FOR THE PERSON TO EXPERIENCE THE LOSS

(A) Being with Others

Being engaged in experiences with others where the loss is a shared experience supports a vital sense of *belonging* or *being connected*. A basic task of the support environment is to insure active participation or involvement in experiences in which the loss is acknowledged, and socially defined. Active participation in any social situations in which the loss is recognized helps the bereaved *realize* the loss. Realizing the loss, or experiencing its *impact* is a first step in grieving. It is a step that continues to resonate throughout the mourning process.

Being as fully involved as possible in the family or other social context surrounding the loss supports the mourning process and the *validity* of the person. Being with other family mourners helps to provide realization, meaning, and connectedness, three vital concerns in supporting the mourning process. Involvement in family interactions around illness and death tends to promote mourning, strength of the self, feelings of belonging and, consequently, the integration of a sense of identity. Involvement with the family provides a bond of nurturance, which, even when there is also family conflict, supports the mourning process.

Being with the family, for example, during a serious or terminal illness of a close family member, to whatever extent is indicated, provides a direct experience and example of other persons dealing with the loss, a sense of meaningful belonging, and an opportunity to directly and concretely experience the loss. The experience of connectedness at important times in the life history of a person, such as the death of loved ones, may be deeply nurturing and supportive of security and self-worth, and help in reckoning with the loss. Even when family connections may be somewhat disturbing, the advantages need to be weighed against the disadvantages, and involvement is likely to be indicated. Enabling the client to participate in family rituals, such as a funeral, may provide especially significant meaning and connectedness. Bearing witness to one's grief in such a social context, nurtures a basic sense of security, identity, and self-worth, and may be deeply meaningful for the rest of the person's life.

(B) Doing Things

Being engaged in activities in which the loss is acknowledged, or being active and doing things that recognize and help process the loss, is useful in mourning. Active involvement provides an experience in which loss is wrapped with meaning and symbolized. Activities of various kinds may be set up for the purpose of supporting the mourning process. Lutcherhand and Murphy (1998), in their book *Helping Adults with Mental Retardation Grieve a Death Loss,* give a menu with suggestions of diverse activities to help facilitate the mourning process, such as drawing a picture of grief feelings, or a picture of the deceased, using a prayer or poem, or an audiotape of meaningful music, enlarging and framing a photo, making a memory box, journaling, making or finding objects that may be reminders of the deceased, and many more. It may be useful for staff and managers to talk together and develop a support plan of interpersonal support strategies and activities.

Rituals are basic cultural language for dealing with changes, and often it is helpful, in supporting the grief of others to facilitate the development of rituals for acknowledging a loss. Developing a ritual should be a very intentional, thoughtful process, so that the bereaved has as fully as possible invested his or her grief in the symbolism of the ritual. *Preparation* for the ritual is an important part of the ritual process. The ritual should be designed as a response to the specific grief needs of the bereaved. For example, if the grieving person is angry or guilty, the ritual might involve asking or seeking forgiveness; or, if the grieving person needs to say goodbye, the ritual may be designed to do this; or, if the need is to secure a sense of continued meaningful connection, a ritual to express this may be developed.

Related to the strong tendency toward compulsivity among persons with mental retardation, ritual may operate as a particularly powerful therapeutic language. Ritual is usually a social event in which the loss is recognized, or some meaningful action symbolically performed, such as saying goodbye. These rituals involve symbolization of the loss and bearing witness to the loss or the act of mourning. But therapeutic rituals may also be private, such as creating and repeating a prayer or another self-caring and self-soothing ritual gesture. A private visit to a gravesite may also be a healing ritual.

While rituals occur at a given moment in time, aspects may be maintained in a continuing way. If a ritual involves hanging pictures on a wall, it may be supportive of the person's grief vulnerability and of a continuing bond with the deceased to frame the pictures and keep them hung on the wall. A site, such as a decorated bulletin board, may be a memorial board where pictures may be kept for all members of the community who have experienced a loss. Continued recognition may be facilitated by setting up a place for mementos. Another example is the planting of a tree in a grief ritual, which will continue as a sacred memorial place. For further discussion of this process the reader may consult Rando's (1993, pp. 313-331) discussion of creating therapeutic bereavement rituals in *Treatment of Complicated Mourning*.

In addition to maximizing active participation in activities that recognize and help to symbolize the loss, the grief helper also aims to maximize opportunities for self expression, and may create activities, such as drawing pictures of feelings, or talking about grief in a group with others, in which the person may express his grief.

SUPPORT THE ADAPTATION NEEDS
OF THE GRIEVING PERSON

When a change occurs a key part of the process of recovering from the loss is *adaptation* to changes that the loss inflicts. Helping the person adjust to change in routines, physical environments, relationships, or other circumstances of their life that are different, is often the most critical part of the adjustment process after a loss. We might say that the mourning process may have retrospective and prospective elements: the retrospective aspects of grief face what is lost, and the prospective aspects look toward the future, and the new situation in which one finds oneself. As we look at the prospective significance of adjustment to change, we should not allow ourselves to devalue the deeply meaningful retrospective aspects; as the positive encouragements and concreteness of adjusting to the new environment may sometimes prompt a support person to do. Adjusting to the new environment will usually have elements of looking back to what is gone, and reckoning with the pain of this.

In the case of Marla we may see how her family provided support of her painful grief over what she lost and support for the process of adjusting to the changed environment at the same time. Marla had lived in the same house since birth. Her mother died when Marla was in her early 30s. A couple of years later her father died. She had been with her mother when she died, calling out to her not to die, and holding her. Then when her father died, Marla was the one who found him. Several siblings, who'd long since left home and had families of their own, stepped in and alternated living with Marla in their parents' home. They did this for about a month, during which time a plan for where Marla would live was worked out. They talked openly with her, supporting her routines, comforting and validating her and providing her with close emotional support for her grief over the death of her parents. Marla and her siblings explored the possibility of keeping her in the home, and worked hard at trying to figure a way to do it. So when the decision was reached that she could not stay at home, Marla, despite being grief-stricken about having to leave home, was in accord with her brothers and sisters in thinking it was necessary. Several siblings were willing to have Marla live with them, and Marla was able to choose who she would live with. Visits to her sister's home were arranged so Marla could look at the room that would be hers and see how she would fix the room up to suit her. A goodbye party for the old house was set up, and pictures taken for a memory book. This situation worked out very well, and one should take it as an ideal example of aspects of a family supporting adjustment.

PREPARATION FOR THE DEATH OF A PRIMARY FAMILY CAREGIVER

Loss of a primary caregiver is a major event in a person's life, and is a concern that many families live with, especially where the primary caregiver is aging, or ill, or otherwise aware of their mortality. The concern is, "What will happen to the person with mental retardation when the primary caregiver dies?"

Preparation for the death of the primary caregiver is often avoided because of anxiety about facing the inevitability of death.

When the primary caregiver faces the fact, and realizes that she[1] is likely to pre-decease the person she cares for, she can then take steps and do some things that will be of supportive value after the death. Having a plan of things to do that will help the person after her death, has the further benefit that it reduces the primary caregiver's anxiety about the future well-being of the person cared for, and may help the primary caretaker with her own life and her own death.

Loss of a primary caregiver means loss of a basic attachment bond and loss of the grounding, security, and familiarity which the bond provides. Loss of a primary caregiver may trigger a grief reaction flooded with feelings such as abandonment, self-blame, anger, loneliness, confusion, and fear about loss of the basic supportive environment. The person may not "get over" the loss, but learn to live with it—the *memory* of the primary caregiver and of their death being an enduringly meaningful connection. Loss of the primary caregiver may mean that other important losses also occur. These include, loss of home; loss of the bond to and security of familiar surroundings, activities, people, and objects; loss of the bond to and security of routines; loss of a whole life in which one's sense of identity and reality is rooted.

By anticipating and preparing for the consequences of her own death the primary caregiver may help ease the way and set up care for the person. The broken attachment to the primary caregiver and to life at home is a loss often difficult to adjust to. Typically, this adjustment process lasts nine months to two or three years, and it may, sometimes, never be a good adjustment. Complicating factors around the death or placement process may extend the adjustment process. Finally, an adjustment may occur while varieties of attachment feelings and bonds endure, where the attachment to the primary caregiver remains, and a deep continuation of aspects of the emotional life and bondedness is at the heart of the person all his or her life. Dennis Klass has, talked about this as a *continuing bond* (Klass, Silverman, and Nickerman, 1996).

---

[1] I believe in and support the equality of men and women. However, I ask the readers to please accept the outdated "he, him, and his" when it appears in my writing reflecting either or both genders. I use these words rather than gender-free language in order to avoid distracting from my essential message for the sake of another, important as that one is.

When one is able to anticipate a change, it helps to have a sense of "knowing" about what is going on, a sense of control in face of a change. It supports an internal *preparation* process that may reduce feelings of being caught off guard, and that provides some anchors to secure the person in the upheaval after the death of the primary caregiver. An important part of the preparation process is finding meaningful and appropriate ways of involving the person in interactions and activities that will be of emotional benefit to him or her after the death of the primary caregiver.

The protocols suggested here are intended to address the psychological needs of the person with mental retardation that may occur after the death of a primary caretaker. A major upheaval of the familiar, predictable, known world the person lives in, and a loss of the security and resources of a relationship in which he is deeply "known" are the general risks addressed by the support guidelines proposed here.

The primary caregiver begins the process of developing a plan by thinking about her concerns and her hopes; and aims to develop a plan of action that addresses the experience of loss, the pain of grief, the vulnerabilities of separation anxiety, and continuity of care issues.

(A) Developing a Plan for the Care of the Person with Mental Retardation After the Caregiver's Death

1. Deciding who will care for the person, and how this will be set up is a big decision. The basic choices are between a family member and a residential service provider. In making the decision the primary caregiver may wish to seek input from family, advocacy groups, and the county mental retardation office. Talking to a counselor may be helpful in making a decision about care and guardianship.

2. If a family member is to be the new caregiver, then, of course, this should be discussed with concern for the needs of all parties, and the person with mental retardation should have maximum involvement in the process. Difficulties that are anticipated should be addressed, so far as possible, beforehand. The primary caregiver should write a fairly comprehensive letter to family members setting out needs and goals, summarizing family discussions and decisions.

3. Placement, before it is a necessity, should also be considered. Placement while the caregiver is still available to help with the

post-placement adjustment process is often a good plan. Furthermore, when a primary caregiver is ill or has died and placement is done in an emergency, the grieving person is faced with multiple losses and adjustments at the same time. And, if placement is needed on an urgent basis then there will most likely be a series of short term placements while waiting for or searching for a long-term placement.

4. The person with mental retardation should be included in all aspects of the planning process as fully as possible. The rule of thumb is maximum possible involvement of the person in the whole process. Involvement is a matter of respect and maximizing autonomy, and may help with adaptation after the loss occurs. Even if the person does not fully understand, including him or her in the process in whatever way possible, is recommended.

5. The primary caregiver knows many things about the needs, habits, patterns of behavior, preferences, things enjoyed, idiosyncrasies, and knows the history of the person with mental retardation. The history of a person may include many different things, such as medical and developmental information, a history of losses, relationships, meaningful experiences, family stories, and many other stories that are part of who the person is.

The information may be written down, together with an account of the caregiver's own feelings, and their relationship with the person. Many different kinds of things may be said in such a document. It is a document that may also be read to and discussed with the person while it is being pulled together and composed, or, for that matter, at any time. It may be thought of as a narrative that accompanies the person on their journey, if he or she moves outside the family, among strangers who will, in a different way, become family. It may be thought of as a resource and a history that supports the person in the future.

6. A part of setting up this care plan is consulting with an attorney. There are important legal issues that need to be taken care of. Attorneys may be located through local advocacy groups, such as the Association For Retarded Citizens (ARC).The legal instruments that need to be discussed with an attorney include a will which makes specific provisions for person with disability and a special needs trust (which is also called a supplemental needs trust, and discretionary trust). The intentional process of setting up guardianship is done in consultation with an attorney. An attorney may also be helpful with regard to social security benefits.

A part of the nuts and bolts of planning is establishing contact with not only local advocacy groups, but also the County Office of Mental Retardation, and any other relevant government agencies.

(B) Develop a Plan of Things To Do in Caregiver's Relationship with the Person that Will Be Helpful to the Person After Caregiver's Death

What can the primary caregiver do in their relationship with the person with mental retardation that will help with the mourning process when the primary caretaker dies?

1. Talking about death, separation, or grief feelings and thoughts may be useful, and may be done in conjunction with discussion of care plans for the person after the death of the primary caregiver. This is also a way of preparing for saying goodbye, which is a very hard part of the relationship, and, often, an important part of the relationship.

Sometimes it is helpful for the caregiver to think about their own anxieties in approaching the subject of their death. These anxieties will tell the caregiver a lot about his or her own feelings about the relationship and the meaning of the loss, and other matters of concern about one's own existence and life. Becoming aware of these feelings is a good place for the primary caregiver to start in deciding how he or she wants to approach this, and what to say.

2. The primary caregiver may tell the person stories about his or herself, about the person, about their relationship, and, most of all, about things they have experienced together, or any stories that may be remembered and nurture a sense of connection. These stories may be written down for the person, for them to read or to be read to them, and for future use. In addition to serving as mnemonic connectors, the stories may serve other functions. If there is concern about self-blame or anger in the relationship, narratives of conflict and *reconciliation* may be useful. The person with mental retardation will then have these stories for support in their grief, to help sustain meaningful memories and contribute to a sense of inner harmony and connectedness.

I recommend that stories be bound up with physical objects, for example, photo albums or memory books or other memory objects. These objects may be constructed together, and looked at and talked about together. Other physical objects, such as something that belongs to the primary caregiver, may also have special emotional meaning associated with them, and these may be given to the person as part of the preparation process or as a bequest. Special objects and special stories help provide connection, meaning and safety.

TEACHABLE MOMENTS

A teachable moment is a time to talk about feelings related to death or other loss, a time to name and describe feelings; or it may be a time to talk about the meaning of death, such as its irreversibility or spiritual beliefs about death. It may be a time to talk about losses that have been experienced; it may be a time to talk about grief ritual, or about what people need when experiencing a loss; it may be a time to elicit misunderstandings and worries and address them.

Whenever a death occurs that is not a significant loss, the event may be taken as an opportunity for death and grief education. When a pet or a plant dies, when a story about death in the news is on a person's mind, or when other persons are bereaved are examples of occasions when death and grief may be addressed. The primary aim of a teachable moment is to advance the normalization and integration of death and loss, and to provide thoughts and concepts that may be useful to the person in personal experiences of loss. Teachable moment interventions also may help make death and loss more familiar and a part of life. Familiarization with facts and with feelings related to death and loss may strengthen the self's ability to accommodate to the reality of losses and provides a cognitive context that may help a person when a death occurs.

Teachable moments may be planned for by having an educational agenda in place, and ready for use when it is timely. Client education is discussed further in the chapter on program development.

ANNIVERSARIES AND HOLIDAY: PERSONAL MEMORIAL DAYS

On the anniversary of a death there may occur what is known as an anniversary reaction. Memory has a remarkable tendency to bring up, at the approach of the anniversary of a death, an affective grief reaction. Memory has an unconscious mental calendar that anticipates the arrival of the anniversary. The grief experience is, in a way, relived. Anniversary reactions are calendar-cued mnemonic spasms, expressions of the enduring presence of a loss that has ceased to be a conscious preoccupation, and a reliving of the emotionally charged aspects of the death. The grief that occurs as the anniversary of a death approaches, similar to grief at other memorial days, such as birthdays and other special days, spontaneously erupts as a memorial to the deceased and as a reliving or a reworking of underlying grief issues. Sometimes the grief reaction will occur without any conscious awareness of the loss. Anniversary grief reactions are normal and meaningful occurrences. Reactions most often occur in an anticipatory way as the anniversary date approaches. And it hardly needs to be said that, clearly, anniversary reactions are *not* "set backs."

An ego supportive approach responds to the anniversary reaction as an opportunity to further work through the loss, and a special time in which to memorialize the deceased and the relationship with the deceased. Looking at memorial objects, such as pictures or objects associated with the deceased, or a visit to persons or places associated with the deceased, such as a grave visit or a family visit, may be helpful. These are ritual remembrances. If the grief that comes up is especially disruptive, or recognized to be related to some chronic underlying grief disturbances, an evaluation by a grief therapist is indicated.

LOIS

Lois is a 37-year-old woman living in a Community Living Arrangement. I met her just before the 11th anniversary of her mother's death. She had become physically violent, destroying property and hitting people. She said, "I feel like nobody loves me. . . . I feel my hands are going to do something I don't want them to do." Every year since her mother's death, as the anniversary approached, she began acting out aggressively. After a couple of months she settled down, and there were no behavioral disturbances until the next anniversary rolled around.

I asked her about feeling that no one loved her. In the course of talking about this she said, "I made her die with my problems." This expression of underlying guilt in her grief pointed to the salient "unresolved" issue that exploded on the scene annually. She felt unloved and rejected by her mother's death, and blamed herself for this. This grief reaction was the recurrence of the regressive undertow in her relationship with her mother. This narcissistic injury of abandonment and self-blame for feeling unloved was not, for Lois, significantly evident at other times during the course of the year. It is as if she had resolved this problem well enough to function well and had no disturbances all the rest of the year, but the anniversary served her unconscious self by acknowledging that this issue was not truly settled for her. Her outburst of rage was an acknowledgment of the injury and reclaimed her anger, which was re-witnessed and remembered as an act of justice and retribution for the injury that continued to be there. When the anniversary of her mother's death approached, the feeling of being unloved and at fault for the death erupted and was expressed by destructive acting out.

When she reflected, ". . . I feel my hands are going to do something I don't want them to do," we can see that she recognized her destructive action, but experienced it as if it were carried out by a separate agent, dissociated, but within her, who was filled with aggression. The anniversary reaction was not an act of her conscious ego, but it came up inside her as an expression of the grief that continued to be there in her continuing relationship with her mother.

She and I talked about her mother and her relationship with her mother; I encouraged her and staff to talk about her mother and her relationship with her mother; and a trip to the cemetery was arranged, and planned as an annual pilgrimage, where she placed flowers at the grave and talked to her mother to seek reconciliation and loving connection. These anniversary interventions reduced the duration and intensity of her aggressive behavior.

THE COLLABORATIVE RELATIONSHIP
BETWEEN GRIEF COUNSELOR/THERAPIST
AND AGENCY OR FAMILY

The relationship between the grief specialist and the primary supportive environment of agencies and families is a collaborative one. It is recommended that the grief specialist and the supportive environment approach their relationship with the expectation of mutual learning. The aim is that the mutual concern about the grief of the person with mental retardation find expression in this relationship and lead, so far as it fits the situation, to a mutually developed treatment plan, carried out by both the grief specialist and the primary supportive environment. This involves planning both what the primary support environment needs to do to support the mourning process, and what the grief therapist needs to do. It may involve sharing of information and support strategies.

The collaborative relationship between the grief counselor/therapist and the supportive environment must be careful to respect privacy needs and support the autonomy of the person, and to guard the confidentiality of the counseling/therapy relationship. But, in certain ways the *client* of the grief counselor/therapist is both the grieving person with mental retardation *and* the support environment in which they live.

The grief counselor/therapist usually needs information from the agency and family in order to assess the grief situation, and ongoing communication about what happens in between sessions is often needed. It is usually best for the person to be present at these discussions. Sometimes written notes on what has happened between sessions may be provided by the agency, and may be read aloud and discussed in the session. For staff to come in at the beginning of a session and discuss what has happened since the last session is often helpful. In some situations staff or family may be in the session for all or part of the time.

The grief specialist may be interested in how the staff responds to and supports the grief behaviors of the person with mental retardation. The support environment, for their part, may wish help from the grief counselor/therapist in strategizing supportive responses to grief behaviors. In developing a support plan the grief specialist may assess the way that the agency staff supports the person's grief, and, if needed, help staff find more supportive responses. The way a person experiences grief is likely to be influenced by how they experience the supportive environment responding to their grief. The grief counselor/therapist helps the support environment understand grief behaviors and develop supportive responses.

In some situations in which a grief counselor/therapist collaborates with an agency, the staff may also be experiencing grief over the death of a client or a staff member. If this is the case, opportunities for staff discussing their own grief should be provided, such as a grief counselor/therapist facilitating a staff meeting where staff may express and share grief issues and build mutual support. The role of the grief counselor/therapist includes nurturing the day-to-day environment of the grieving person with mental retardation.

In the context of the collaborative relationship between the consulting grief counselor/therapist and the agency, agency needs for program development, such as discussed in this book may be evaluated.

GRIEF SUPPORT INTERVENTIONS
FOR A RESIDENCE

What to Do When a Peer is Dying

When a peer in a residential, work, or social group is seriously ill and dying the facility needs to evaluate the impact on others in the group. Information about the person's illness should usually be provided, and questions encouraged and answered. Opportunities for group and one-on-one discussions of facts and feelings may be provided about the illness and its symptoms, hospitals , death, being sick, the sick or dying person, anxieties about oneself, distressing memories that pop up in reaction to the situation, or whatever is on person's minds and in their feelings. Among other things that may be done are group prayers for the sick person, or conducting a ritual, such as lighting candle, or sending a group card to the hospital.

When a peer dies the peer group should be provided opportunities to talk about and ritualize the loss. Every effort should be made to arrange for those who wish to attend the funeral, to do so, and a peer group memorial event, that may include inviting the family, may also be planned.

Whenever a loss affects a peer group, opportunities should be provided for members of the group to have a facilitated group meeting to discuss the experience.

When a person dies, it is meaningful to wait a respectful period of time before filling their residential slot. It helps other residents because the person's room and things maintain a physical reminder of the deceased person. As well as being a meaningfully respected place where death occurred and that belonged to the deceased (it is *their* room), it is place that provides a touchstone for peer grief. Filling the bed signals "moving on," and this should not be done too soon. Sometimes a few weeks is sufficient, other times it may take longer until the residents are ready for someone else to be sleeping in the bed that the deceased housemate had slept in.

The very need to fill the bed may sometimes be brought into a group discussion.

It may help the mourning process if, when possible, the decision to fill the bed explicitly takes meaningful account of the wishes and feelings of residents. And, just before the deceased person's place is prepared for a new resident is a good time for a transition ritual and saying goodbye, again, to the person. The ritual might be doing something to say goodbye to the room or bed as the room or bed of the deceased, and something to ready it to welcome the new person.

Intense Grief Disrupts a Residence

One resident's grief from a death or other loss may affect the life of a whole residence. Typically aggressive acting out will affect others, and may impact on others, and affect their psychological well being. In the case that follows we see an example of how the grief of one resident affected another resident.

Jean, a grieving woman became intensely jealous when, on weekends, the mother of another resident, Cindy, came to pick her up. Jean told her that she was a bad person for having a mother, and aggressively condemned and insulted her. Cindy began to feel it was wrong to go with her mother. She got angry with her mother for being alive, and started to refuse to see her mother. She was depressed and angry, and needed staff support and validation and a brief psychotherapeutic intervention.

REFERENCES

Klass, D., Silverman, P., & Nickman, S. L. (1996). *Continuing bonds.* Philadelphia: Taylor & Francis.

Luchterhand, C., & Murphy, N. (1998). *Helping adults with mental retardation grieve a death loss.* Philadelphia: Accelerated Development Press.

Rando, T. (1993). *Treatment of complicated mourning.* Champaign: Research Press.

CHAPTER 3

The Language of Grief
in Persons with
Mental Retardation

INTRODUCTION TO THE BEHAVIORAL
LANGUAGE OF GRIEF

The primary grief language of persons with mental retardation is
behavioral. Sometimes, when behavior speaks, the meaning of what
is communicated is clear, sometimes it is opaque, and sometimes it,
or we, are dense, and no meaning is disclosed. Even when the actions
which express grief are self-evidently meaningful, there is, as we
shall see, usually more going on than meets the eye at first. We shall
see that sometimes, as we are attentive to expressions of grief over
time, our understanding of what the grief language is expressing
changes. These changes basically point out how we are part of
process, and that if we regard our own perceptions of meaning as
hypotheses, rather than certainties, we are more able to fine tune,
and deepen our understanding, and so be better able to respond
supportively. No hypothesis about what is expressed in grief
language ought to have a standing any greater than its capacity
to keep us well attuned to the pain it expresses.

The grief language of persons with mental retardation discloses
intellectual capacities that are no less powerful, complex, subtle,
disturbing, deep, and spiritual than found in the more discursive and
dialectical grief language of persons without mental retardation.
In this chapter and in Chapter 4 on psychological concerns and
complications, cases will be presented with the aim of showing the

expressive and communicative language of grief in persons with mental retardation, demonstrating how this language expresses grief and how to listen to it.

The starting place for understanding the behavioral language of the grieving person with mental retardation is to recognize that a particular grief behavior is a symbolic expression of grief; or, put otherwise, we need to recognize that grief distress is being expressed, and respond supportively. This is often the case in uncomplicated grief. It is merely a matter of observing a behavior, asking oneself what is being expressed, or what is the behavior *saying*, and constructing a narrative that gives a sufficient or good enough account of the *meaning* of the grief behavior. In this context an operational definition of "good enough account" is that it tells us what is going on, or works as a starting place for developing a plan of supportive response, a plan that may adjust, as needed, to changes in our understanding of what the person's grief language is expressing.

First and foremost, to the extent that the person experiences his or herself to be understood, significant grief support is being provided. Grief support interventions by a grief counselor/therapist or by the supportive environment are, primarily, responses to the behavioral language of the grieving. Mere empathic recognition of expressions of grief, in whatever way this recognition is given, is the most basic supportive and therapeutic aspect of helping the person with mental retardation mourn. Facilitating the mourning process is simply being attuned to and responding to the behavioral language of grief. The communicative process between expressions of grief and the supportive environment's receptivity and acceptance is an interaction in which the grief process is facilitated.

Expressions of grief are a language, an expressive-communicative grief language. Mourning is often defined as the expression of grief, that is, the social or communicative act of expressing grief. The expressive language of grief *is* an act of mourning. Even though mourning is, in another, deeply psychological sense, very private, it does exists in a context of social interaction, where the environment's responses to the behavioral language of grief becomes part of the mourning process. The language of grief among persons with mental retardation initiates an exchange which is an important part of the construction of the meaning of a loss as it occurs in the mourning process.

The language of grief in persons with mental retardation, with verbal as well as non-verbal persons, is, primarily, an expressive language, a body language, a sometimes purely performance language. The language of grief is an enactment of grief. Grief is expressed in a behavioral drama. Let us look at a few examples of how behavior expresses, shows, and enacts specific grief thoughts or feelings.

NICHOLAS

Nicholas' grief behavior is a clear and intense expression of the initial reaction to the death of a loved one. In this account we see how demonstratively and straightforwardly his behavior enacts the psychodynamics of his grief.

On May 27, 1984 John Woestendiek reported in the Philadelphia Inquirer, *in an article called "The Unwitting Revolutionary of Pennhurst," the story of Nicholas Romeo. The story recounted the horrific fate of Nicholas who was placed in Pennhurst, a state institution for persons with mental retardation, as a result of a very intense grief reaction. The story was reported at the time that Pennhurst was being shut down, telling how the abuse that Nicholas and others suffered led to the closing of Pennhurst.*

Nicholas had arrived at Pennhurst in the deep throes of grief after his father's death. The story begins with an account of Nicholas' initial reactions as he realized that his father was gone. Woestendiek wrote: "In the days that followed [his father's death], Nick, his brown eyes bouncing back and forth between looks of anger, frustration and fear, would run from room to room of the row house, groaning when he couldn't find his father. He would grab his mother's hand, pull her out of the house and lead her to all the places Frank [his father] had taken him."

As he became aware that his father was not to be found, he panicked. "He screamed, and broke things. He kicked and slapped, bit his hand and banged his head against the wall—things he had done only once in while in the past. . . ." He was out of control. Twelve days after his father's death, Nicholas was placed at Pennhurst State School and Hospital, where he was brutalized and he deteriorated.

We can see in Nicholas' behavior his awareness that his father is not there. As he goes from place to place, he is searching for him. The searching says, "Where is he?" As he fails to find him anywhere, the reality of his being gone becomes more certain, and Nicholas's expression of grief becomes more aggressive and intense. His father is nowhere to be found. This is enacted as a dramatic, direct, and very powerful language of realization and anxiety. The increasing panic of his searching expresses both the awareness that his father is gone, and his being overwhelmed by this knowledge. Panic is his grief reaction.

This behavior is a fairly self-evident grief language. It exhibits the specific psychological process of reaction to a loss. The searching and yearning for his father is a normal grief reaction. What his grief language expresses, and what is disturbing, is the intensity of *his searching and yearning, and the intensity of the meaning and the affect of his grief. The intensity of his language acts out and communicates his grief. The intensity of his reaction is so shocking, and it is difficult to put oneself in his shoes, and try to grasp the grief that is expressed in this panic. Yearning is hardly the right word for the intense urgency he expresses. The affective intensity expressed is a key part of the language, expressing traumatization by the literal enactment of intensity. His choreographic language performs his experience of grief, as a physical and forceful abandonment or separation panic. It is a language of terror and helplessness, a dawning fear that his father is gone, that all is lost, and whatever overwhelming significance this holds for Nicholas. His community could not tolerate the intensity of his grief reaction and "put him away."*

Woestendiek's simple description of Nicholas' behavior is a grief narrative. His writing puts into words what Nicholas has expressed in action. Woestendiek perceives, as we do in reading his account, that Nicholas' behavior is an expression of grief. Nicholas' language is a behavioral language, in which the narrative is not expressed in words, but in a dramatic expression of grief, in which abandonment or separation panic seem to occur and to be performed in an expressive act. His behavior is the physical externality of his internal experience of loss. His insistent, concrete, very direct, and affectively charged action language forcefully signifies his grief. Nicholas' language kinetically and graphically enacts his thought, or, more accurately, is his thought.

Searching and yearning, which Bowlby's (1980) grief theory describes as separation anxiety, is, here, an unmitigated separation panic in Nicholas. Searching and yearning actions may provide, through the power of enacting the hope that his father will be found, a measure of control even as the performance/realization of out of control desperation leads to a breakdown of searching and yearning into despair. Hope and despair drive his grief until the hope is crushed, and he is overwhelmed by fear and despair. He fell into this deep hole, and his shattered self never recovered.

Nicholas needed a strong supportive environment in which it was safe to experience his grief, and in which his panicked self's terrified behaviors were understood as grief that, in the first place, only needed safety, comfort, and patience. His powerful expression of grief communicated the intensity of his anxiety, and triggered a reaction in his support community in which it was believed that he could not be managed. A key part of the grief therapist's intervention in such a situation would be to support his environment in tolerating and creating safety for his grief.

DORIS

Doris had temper tantrums whenever she was told something that she took to be a criticism, or when she perceived someone else getting attention. She was extremely sensitive to feeling criticized and abandoned, and tended to feel insulted, and expressed this through fits of rage. Usually the triggering situation was evident, though not always.

Staff at her residence thought that these "acting out" behaviors may have been a grief reaction to her mother's death, which had occurred four years earlier, and precipitated Doris' residential placement. There had been, after her mother's death, a very angry initial grief period that lasted about two years. Since then there had been a number of episodes in which she was angry and withdrawn. The intensity and frequency of these episodes had subsided, and for many months she had not expressed any distress. Then, intense outbursts started up again. It was at this time that she was referred for treatment.

In assessing this situation, the place to start was with her behavior. What was her behavior expressing? The behavior was an expression of rage. But, what was she enraged about? We took a closer look at the triggers *for her outbursts. As already noted, the triggers were: 1) being told what to do, and 2) when someone else got attention, though there were also times when we could not identify a trigger event. Both of these evident trigger events threatened her. When she was told what to do, she felt her autonomy threatened, and she felt demeaned and diminished by this; and, this was associated with her* mother. When someone else got attention, Doris felt abandoned, which was a feeling also associated with her mother, and closely related to feeling like she was being controlled by others, that is, it also made her feel like she was nothing. Both situations evoked a sense of wounded dependence. Both being told what to do and someone else getting attention were narcissistic injuries that she experienced particularly in the dependency aspect of her relationship with her mother. These injuries had, it now appeared, been at the core of her grief over her mother's death.

Doris' grief language took her feeling toward her mother out on others, or experienced it in situations with others. She felt, in her experiences with others, the grief injury of "her mother narcissistically wounding her." She had, herself, no thought of her mother when feeling slighted by others, but it was her feeling this relationship undertow with her mother, the way she missed her mother so strongly, that provoked the replaying or re-experiencing of this narcissistic injury in other relationships in her life since her mother died. Missing her mother, she also needed, I suggest, a reconciliation with her mother; she re-enacted the pain from the relationship with her mother that she was left to deal with. Her grief over her mother's death expressed, then, a need for reckoning with her relationship with her mother. Her grief over her mother's death was an exacerbation of her undercurrent pain in this close relationship. And she had been, since her mother's death, in the grip of this pain; she was able to put it aside for periods of time, but the injury was persistent and would not leave her at peace. It was in her, as her narcissistic "oversensitivity" to loss of autonomy and abandonment.

Doris needed to settle accounts with her mother. I thought that there was a quality to her repeating this injury again and again, each time leading to apology and reconciliation, that comforted her, though the comfort was never long lasting. She was continuing the relationship with her mother through reliving feelings of rejection, abandonment, anger, and reconciliation. The narrative of her acting out included the whole sequence of interactions with residential support staff, that started with an injury to self and led to a reconciliation with staff. As noted, the repeated reconciliations were comforting and helpful, but were not sufficient to heal the injury.

Treatment gave her recognition and validation in her feelings of rejection, abandonment, and anger, and in her seeking reconciliation. Treatment aimed to help her identify the feelings and affirmed her need to express these feelings. Treatment also aimed at supporting staff in understanding her behavior, and in coping with their frustrations in response to her behavior. Over an extended course of grief therapy, the violent eruptions of protest over a narcissistic injury more or less dissolved into a personality trait, in which she took pleasure in criticizing others. She was no longer in distress, and her criticisms of other persons was a mild behavior, recalcitrant to further treatment.

JAMIE

Jamie's father had visited him weekly. Then, after Thanksgiving weekend, he stopped showing up. There was no contact from Jamie's family to tell him that his father had died. He was just gone, and a very dependable, predictable pattern of relationship and Sunday routine was broken. At Christmas of that same year his family brought him home, and told him that his father was dead.

Staff reports that after this Jamie was OK, and seemed to barely miss his father. Then, as the year anniversary of his father's death approached, Jamie began packing his bag, putting on his coat, and sitting by the doorway waiting for his father. Soon, he was ready all the time, wearing his coat, walking around and sleeping at night with his bag packed. The language was clearly saying, "I am waiting for my father."

Was Jamie waiting out of not understanding that his father was dead, or what dead was? Based on my conversation with him about heaven, which I'll give an account of in a moment, I believe he got the idea that dead meant gone. I think his behavior was a delayed grief reaction; he was expressing thoughts and feeling about his father's absence. As the anniversary of the last time Jamie had seen his father approached, he began to miss his father in an intense and compelling way.

It is clear that he was expressing, "I am waiting for my father." That is what he dramatized. And this seems to have meant, "I miss my father." But beyond that, it was unclear if he was saying, "Daddy, where are you?", or "I know you are not coming, but I refuse to believe or accept that," or, "Now that my father is gone, why isn't anyone else in my family coming to visit me and take me out?!" The action itself was a very clear dramatization of "I am waiting for my father," and probably also saying, "I miss him," but beyond this headline, it was not clear exactly what the story was.

All Jamie said was, "No show." He said this whenever anyone asked him what he was doing with his bag packed, his coat on and standing by the door. While this could be taken many ways, I felt he was putting it this way to justify to the person who asked him what he was doing. In effect, then, he is saying, "He hasn't come" in order to explain to the person asking why he was waiting. Or, by saying the words "no show" he was just telling the questioner that he was waiting for his father, period. But, whatever, these words may have said about his grief and his wish for his father to appear, they do not tell us anything that his behavior hadn't said more powerfully. The behavior, in this case, however, is only a starting place in understanding, or in helping him realize, what he is saying.

I asked Jamie where his father was. He pointed upward, and said, "Die, in heaven with Jesus." He seemed, I thought, to understand that his father had died, and he had, from religious stories, a narrative to say where he was. Sometimes he pronounced the words "die" and "heaven" while he moved his hand slowly circling in front of his face, like he was winding up, with his index finger pointing up, and looking at me. Then, suddenly he'd thrust his arm upward, his finger pointing like he was pointing up further than we could see. His head cocked backwards, and his eyes turned upward, gazing at the place he was pointing to. The whole gesture was done with a dramatic flair, and expressing a strong intention of making a point. Jamie was locating death, pointing out the place where his father was. Someone had, no doubt, told him about heaven, but the way he pointed it out to me expressed, more importantly, his own experience with and thought about death.

Then one day, enacting this for me, as he often did, Jamie added another segment to the performance. At the climax of the story, intently gazing upward to heaven, he turned, and looked back at me, carefully shaped his mouth into an oval, and with a tone of enormous surprise or astonishment or realization, but in a very controlled way, said, "Ooooooooohhh!" He said this in a manner that he was telling me something or pointing something out—not that he had just made an observation, but that I should realize something, that I might make this observation. His striking gesture said there was something very significant I should notice. I took off my glasses. We were face to face. Our noses were touching. Jamie took off his glasses. I did not know what "Ooooooooohhh!" meant, and decided to respond as if he had *told me that he was expressing a realization that his father was dead. Maybe he was simply saying, "I realize my father is dead!" or "I do realize that my father is dead!" Even so, I felt he needed me to realize it with him. I contorted my face into an exaggerated expression of sadness, I said, "sad!" He imitated me, made a sad face and said "sad." We repeated this a number of times. I looked him in the eye, gently shook my head up and down and said "sad." We had created a narrative built upon and continuing his "bags packed by the door" dramatization. Simply our talking about his father's death, and talking about it on his terms, more than any of specific interventions, may have been helpful. Our jointly created and enacted drama operated therapeutically for him.*

Jamie's pivotal communication to me in this conversation was his saying "Oooooooooohhh!," but I have only a limited understanding of what he may have been expressing, that is, that it had to do with his father's death. There is a possibility he was telling me about something that was utterly unbelievable. Perhaps, it was about the shock of the utter otherness of death, saying to me something like, "So, do you see now the shock that persists inside me when I realize my father is dead?" or was he saying "I cannot realize that he is not ever really coming back," or "I cannot believe that he is not ever really coming back." Or, was it really a religious revelation about death that I missed completely in my response to him. He was commenting on something he experienced to be, and wanted me to recognize to be, very remarkable and significant. While I am still in the dark about what this really was, this conversation was a moment between us, a pregnant and symbolically powerful moment that seemed to facilitate the mourning process.

In addition to our sessions, I recommended to staff that a plan be made to go to Jamie's father's grave; that family be included in the planning and execution of the visit to the fullest extent; that family be encouraged to express their emotions at the grave with Jamie; that the visit be planned as a ritual event, with words addressed to his father, and a symbolic gesture such as bringing something to the grave to give his father, or other symbolic acts; that photos of the visit be taken, and included in his life story book; and that family be encouraged to visit him more frequently. The next week I invited Jamie's sister to the session, and plans were made for Jamie to visit the gravesite. Soon afterwards he unpacked his bags and stopped waiting for his father at the doorway.

PERRY

About nine months after his father's death, Perry, who lived at home with his mother and worked in a sheltered workshop, began leaving work in the middle of the day, and took the train to the station nearest his home, where his father used to pick him up every day. He would sit there, and wait for his father to come pick him up, as he had always done. About the same time that he started leaving work early every day, he also began having angry outbursts. Perry's grief language clearly expressed that he was missing his father. On the day of his father's death he had waited for him at the train station, and he had never come. Perry had waited hours that cold December day, and his father never came. Finally, a neighbor came and got him.

His father had been his primary caretaker. His father took him to the fire house and to his other neighborhood hangouts. They were always together. But, Perry had been OK for many months after his father's death. Why had this grief behavior been delayed? At first, when I addressed this question, there was no answer. But, many months after Perry and I started talking, his mother gave me some information explained the timing of his reaction, and also helped me to understand the core issue in his grief reaction.

A few months before the grief behavior of going to the train station had started, Perry's mother had begun to fall apart, and express increasing frustration with him. She was overwhelmed by her responsibility to care for Perry alone. She was very ambivalent, and repeatedly threatened to "put him away." She was enacting and communicating to him abandonment and the devastation of his security. With this information my understanding of what Perry was expressing changed. I now assumed that after his father's death, he continued to feel safe and secure enough with his mother, and that the emergence of grief behaviors, months after his death, signaled his feeling that his immediate world, that is, his mother, was collapsing around him. His waiting at the train station seemed to be saying to his father, "Help! Mom is upset and angry and it has me feeling scared. Dad, I need you! Come home and help me!"

Treatment then shifted to focus on supporting his mother's coping and on helping Perry handle the stress of his anxiety vis-a-vis his mother.

REFERENCE

Bowlby, J. (1980). *Loss: Sadness and depression.* Vol. 3 of *Attachment and Loss.* New York: Basic Books.

CHAPTER 4

Psychological Concerns and Complications

INTRODUCTION TO PSYCHOLOGICAL CONCERNS AND COMPLICATIONS

"Complicated grief" is a term that is created to avoid pathologizing the more disturbing expressions of grief, yet it is often used to mean grief that is not normal, that is, pathological grief. From time to time maladaptive or self-destructive grief, or the intensity or persistence of a grief reaction may seem to call for a judgment that these complications of grief *are* deviations from a norm: the "norm" being less disturbing or less complicated grief. The tendency for clinical evaluation of grief to organize around a norm and deviance from a norm, is, at bottom, I think, a strategy to cordon off anxiety about how disturbing and complicated death and loss are, or how much an underlying trauma of human existence and mortality is denied by instituting norms.

The very pain of grief is itself complicated and may be very intense; and self-destructive aspects appear, at times, to be inherent in grief itself. Attempts to make a clear distinction between normal and complicated grief always fall short, though there is deep urge among grief theorists, in society generally, and in most individuals to make this distinction, and to "know" what is normal and what is not. But, I think this "knowledge," is, strictly speaking, a form of self-deception, and, really, does not serve any supportive or clinical goal. It may, further, be an impediment in the treatment of the most disturbing and persistent grief.

For some persons, agency or family support is not enough, and the services of a grief counselor/therapist are needed. But, in order to identify a person who may benefit from such an intervention, there is no need to make a distinction between normal and not normal grief. Sometimes a grief disturbance may feel like too much for a family or agency, or the grief behavior my signal intense distress, aggression or depression—expressed in a way that arouses the concern of the supportive environment. Then, an evaluation by a grief counselor/ therapist is indicated. Then again, it may be helpful to consult with a grief specialist for an evaluation whenever a loss occurs.

In this chapter I have identified expressions of grief that seem to me to demonstrate key psychological features of the experience of grief in persons with mental retardation. The descriptions of the language of grief and of the psychological pathways of grief presented in the cases that follow are intended to stimulate thinking about the psychology of grief in persons with mental retardation, as much as providing an outline of basic trends in their mourning process.

The discussions of clinical material in this chapter are more theoretical than other parts of this book, and, may be difficult for some readers who may prefer to skip this chapter, but I think that there is a need to provide this kind of theoretical account in order to demonstrate the psychodynamics of the grief of persons with mental retardation, and to place these grief reactions within the spectrum of human grief, generally.

COMPULSIVITY, PERSEVERATION AND RITUALIZATION: PREVENTING CHANGE

Compulsivity, and the compulsive phenomena of perseveration and ritualization, are often very powerful forces in persons with mental retardation. With regard to grief, two key factors are: 1) that the distress of grief may heighten compulsivity, and 2) that compulsivity slows or brings to a halt the progressive trajectory of mourning. Compulsivity occurs normally in reaction to loss among persons with mental retardation, and calls our attention to the grief distress that is occurring. Persons with mental retardation are particularly disrupted by change, and compulsivity is a primary defense against this.

Fluctuations in compulsivity may be read as a distress barometer of grief. Compulsivity tends to intensify in reaction to distressing experiences that threaten to overwhelm the self, so that increased compulsivity is a *distress signal*. In grief among persons with mental retardation there may be a persistently heightened compulsivity. Compulsivity is an immediate response to a change occurring that challenges adaptation, and that is resisted. A primary mode of resistance to change in human psychological functioning is compulsive repetition. It functions to attempt to maintain cohesion and hold the self together, though it is also a sign that the self is experiencing itself to be in danger of disintegrating. By repeating the same, again and again, it seeks to prevent change, even while it expresses anxiety about change. Increased compulsivity is both a bulwark against disintegration *and* a signal of disintegration. Compulsivity conserves and coheses experience. It holds things together. It is centrifugal, reinforcing itself by its action. And, when order and security are experienced to be endangered, compulsivity tends to increase, signaling increased disintegration anxiety. Compulsivity operates to conserve the status quo, and prevent the *experience* of loss, though the more intense the compulsivity the more one experiences loss as disintegration anxiety. Persons with mental retardation display compulsivity in concrete, graphic, and immediate ways that suggest the powerful role, in responses to change, of a disintegration-of-self anxiety.

Processing loss requires relinquishing some compulsivity. It involves a breakdown of a familiar, predictable structure of everyday life and a weakening of the relative security and repetitious routines associated with who or what is lost. And it involves anxiety about the loss of self-cohesion.

Initiated by the shock of loss, by trauma at the core of change, grief may threaten the safety provided by knowing concretely the world one lives in, and in which the self experiences itself, and is anchored. Compulsivity aims to bind anxiety, to seal off the flux of death that is present in the shock of change, of loss, or of a relationship broken by death. A compulsive undertow of human thought process functions as a defense against psychic trauma, *and* there may be a particular vulnerability to the traumatic core of grief among persons with mental retardation. As the internal turmoil of traumatic loss anxiety veers towards getting out of control, compulsivity intensifies. And as the self experiences itself in danger of being overwhelmed and annihilated by this anxiety, it is prone to infuse compulsivity with aggression. The intensity of this anxiety and the rigidity of the compulsive defense against it make a process of relinquishing compulsive control and adapting to change much more difficult.

HAROLD .

Harold reacted to an anxiety aroused by his father's death with an obsessive thought. He was preoccupied with the image of his dead father in a coffin which he had seen at the funeral. This image generated a thought in him, which, however, he was unable to think. It was too horrible, though it held him in a kind of fascination. It was this tension between the image of his dead father and the unthinkable thought associated with this image that triggered his obsessive thought. He couldn't think the thought, and he couldn't stop thinking it.

Harold walked up to everyone he met and talked about his father in a coffin, lying there, not moving. He said to me, "My father is lying in the coffin?" He was asking a question, but he did not know the question he was asking. He was simply describing what he had seen— his father in a coffin, dead, and he was asking a question about it.

I, also, did not know what the question was that he was asking. Was he saying something like, "Is my father really dead?"; or, "Dead? a dead body?, my father dead? what is dead, my god, what is dead?"; or, "My father died, I miss him unbearably, and I am confused about his not being here." Whatever he was asking, it was the image of his dead father that he obsessed over, that troubled him, and that signified something incomprehensible to him.

Sometimes, when he said his father was "lying in the coffin," he added the phrase, "not moving." "My father is lying in the coffin, not moving?" Adding the words "not moving" suggested something about death struck him. Thanatologists sometime call this way that death presents itself to the living as the "non-functionality" of the dead body. Harold perceived and articulated a concern that there was something about the immobility of his father's body that he could not comprehend, or that signified something he did not understand. His concern over the lack of movement of the dead body of his father, which is, certainly, the key observable feature of death, suggested that the anxiety and the question it drove him to repeat over and over may be something like "a body that once moved and now does not move? a dead body? how can a living body change into a dead body? what is dead?" He was obsessed with this image of death.

Harold's obsession with the image of his father's dead body, however, was not accompanied by any other behavioral disturbances, suggesting that his obsession was operating on a primarily cognitive level. We may assume that there was fear here, but there was no particular evidence of fear. His obsessional thought about his father's dead body was, no doubt, a defense against the change from living to being dead that presented the very possibility of death as the lifelessness of his father's body that he witnessed. "How could a living person now be not able to move?" was not a medical or empirical question of any kind, but an expression of existential shock. We see here how Harold puzzled over a basic experience of change, which did not have to do with a change he himself experienced, like changes in his daily routine, residence, bodily sensations, but was pointedly a thought about the death of a person.

DEPENDENCE/ATTACHMENT

When a loss of relationship in which there is a high degree of dependence occurs, there is risk that a continuing and heightened dependency need may occur in grief—triggered, frustrated, and exacerbated by the absence of an attachment object. Broken attachment to a dependency object may lead to intense longing and missing, abandonment anxiety and self-blame as complications of grief. Attachment bonds to the lost love object are at risk of persisting as narcissistic injuries, and may be expressed by aggression or increased compulsivity; or, positive and negative aspects of the bond that has been broken may be enacted in other relationships in which the grief injury tends to get re-experienced. When there has been, side by side with the attachment, a sufficient degree of individuation, or some other adaptive strengths, the loss of an attachment bond may not lead to a complicated broken attachment-bond grief. But, dependency in a relationship is a risk factor for complex reactions that might include: 1) separation anxiety, loss of self-worth, loss of self-confidence, loss of concrete security, etc.; 2) protest behaviors over this loss; and 3) defensive moves, aiming to block (a) abandonment and helplessness anxiety, and (b) guilt over the loss.

Relationships with persons on whom one is dependent are, over the course of the relationship, especially vulnerable to narcissistic injury. The history of the relationship is prone to be strewn with disappointments, frustrations and anger, self-deprecation, and self-blame. When the relationship is broken, injuries rooted in the stresses of a dependency relationship are liable to be activated as a grief reaction. When depression is present in a dependency relationship, then the risk, when the relationship is broken, is an exacerbation of the depression.

Dependency relationships often generate ambivalence, complex mixtures of opposite feelings. And grief over a broken dependency relationship may heighten the opposition or tension between love and hate, attachment and abandonment, good and bad, etc. Where there are strong dependency attachments, autonomy is likely to be more fragile, and might become difficult to maintain when the attachment object is lost.

When there is an experience of being violated emotionally, physically or sexually, especially when the violation occurs within a relationship that is also a source of a sense of safety, identity and being at home, then the risks of a particularly difficult grief are significant. When there are complications in the relationship with a dependency object, the person is prone to be preoccupied with those relationship problems. Difficult grief after the death of a loved one may be expressed in re-enacting the ambivalence in other relationships, and in acts of aggression.

In the dependency relationship, the person upon whom one is dependent becomes an integral part of one's self-regulation, self-concept, and self-worth. The loss may weaken the security, integrity and cohesion of the self.

CHAD

Several years after the death of his Aunt Lois, Chad began compulsively saying he was going to visit her. At the beginning of treatment this was taken to be an indication that he did not understand that she had died, but it turned out to have to do with very uncomplicated attachment issues.

In assessing the situation I learned that the happiest memories that Chad had of his family were the visits to his Aunt Lois' vacation home, where family gatherings had occurred for many years, and where he had continued to visit, long after his parents died, until his aunt died, a few years prior to the emergence of this behavior.

Visits to her cabin in the woods had come to stand for the attachment and security he had felt in his family. Long after Chad's mother's death, his mother's sister Lois, continued to be there, and he made annual visits to her cabin. She loved him and he looked forward to seeing her, and it was the setting of his last experiences of the bondedness of his family.

Chad's relationship with his family had been, and continued to be, a basic part of who he was, his sense of identity. For years after his parents' death, other relatives, and then staff, had continued to take him to his Aunt Lois' cabin every summer until she died. When he was told that she had died staff thought that he understood this. When he started talking about visiting her, there was, as I noted, concern that he did not understand that she had died. The initial treatment goal was helping him realize that she was gone, but it quickly became clear that the "grief behavior" did not have to do with his not realizing that she was dead and gone, but with his missing her and his family.

At the time Chad was brought for grief therapy, he had become preoccupied with talking about going to his Aunt Lois' cabin. He was constantly saying, "I think I might be going to the Poconos this summer." This was sometimes followed by his talking about various aunts and cousins. He was preoccupied with these memories, and talked about it constantly. Staff repeatedly told him that his aunt had died, but he was oblivious to these reality checks, and persisted in saying he thought he might be going to his aunt's cabin. Staff was concerned and took from the constant repetition of his talking about seeing his aunt, and his intermittent explosive outbursts, that he was experiencing a grief problem.

His use of the phrase "I think I might be going" is an interesting and meaningful way of speaking. He spoke this as if he were making a wish. He often expressed wishes as realities, such as, "No, Aunt Lois is not dead. I'll be seeing her this summer," or "I just saw her a few weeks ago." His speech seemed to be part protest and denial, and part an insistent wish, in which he used language as a kind of magic, hoping to make something happen simply by speaking. And, while his saying, "No, she is not dead" had seemed to express denial, as I talked to Chad I came to think that it was not expressing his failure to realize that she was dead, but was a retort to being told she was dead. The thought seemed more to be an assertion of the validity of his wanting to visit his aunt's cabin.

Chad's talking about visiting his aunt was an expression of: 1) missing his family and 2) wanting to get staff to comply with his wish to visit his aunt's cabin, needing, I gather, to experience the bond to his family and the nurturance of this bond. He was making a request, "Please take me to my aunt's cabin." The "please take me" was expressed in such a passive, indirect way, more like trying to conjure it up by saying it out loud, that it was not recognized to be the expression of a desire. But, while it was not a direct assertion of his will, it was an effort to command, by persistence, that he be taken. His periodic outbursts were not simply a complaint that his family was gone, but expressed his frustration that no one seemed to understand what he was saying. Treatment was, mostly, a process in which, eventually, after several weeks, I gathered that he missed his family and wanted to visit his aunt's cabin; and then I arranged for this to happen.

Chad's manner of speech reflected his dependency on others who, too often, did not hear him, and so he internalized this and often spoke as if no one was listening to him, and he was invisible—murmuring passive, wish-making incantations into the thin air. When he said he wanted see to his aunt, he half looked away while he spoke. He spoke very hesitantly, but I thought there was also, tucked inside his timidity, an emphatic confidence and determination that it was going to happen. The intensity of Chad's longing was mainly evident in the insistence of his talking about it—all the time, and in his occasional angry outbursts; otherwise his affect was flat and often gave the impression that he was distractedly musing out loud to himself.

At our second session, still operating with the goal of helping him realize that his aunt had died, but having come to suspect that he did know she was not alive, I said to him, "When you say that Aunt Lois is alive, you mean you wish she were alive." I looked at him, and he looked at me. In a reciprocally questioning gaze, we just looked at each other for what seemed like a long time. I said, "You know she has died." He preoccupied himself with something while I talked, as if he were ignoring me. Then, he leaned toward me, slowly and deliberately, and whispered, loud as a whisper can be, and in a very emphatic way, "Yes!" His manner of speech was that he was not just answering my question, but telling me something very important, something I did not realize that he was pointing out to me. There was no passivity as he spoke directly to me and forcefully. His tone of voice seemed to say, "Do you get it?" And, as he said "yes," I felt that we were engaged in some sort of conspiracy together, that we had just entered into a pact, and that everything was now O.K. It was then that I realized that of course he knew she was dead. It was me who didn't know that he knew. "Of course I know" is what he was saying to me. He knew Aunt Lois was dead, of course. It was then I realized that he was only asking to go visit her cabin. And, now, it seemed so obvious. My experience was that he delivered the word "yes" to me with an extraordinarily focused intention to communicate his thought, and, for all his not being heard so much of the time, and having poor communication skills, he demonstrated, in this instance, a knack for expressing himself.

A trip was arranged. With his lone remaining uncle and a staff person, Chad went on a journey to his aunt's cabin. He went to remember and to say hello and to say goodbye, and to bring the memory of the visit back home with him. The presenting "problem behaviors" ceased.

AMBIVALENCE

Ambivalence is feeling two opposite ways at the same time. As noted in the previous section, ambivalence is a particular risk in relationships with a high degree of dependency or in complicated attachments. The vulnerability of the dependent person tends to increase both negative and positive feelings. When a person is dependent on another the positive attachment bond is likely to be strong, but narcissistic vulnerability to disappointments, abandonment anxiety, feeling hurt, frustration, resentment, anger, and hatred is also likely to be strong, along with feelings of self-devaluation and anger at oneself. When the relationship is broken, grief is prone to be difficult and complicated by an activation of tension between, on the one hand, longing for the bond and missing the deceased, and, on the other, narcissistic frustration, negativity, hurt, and angry feelings. This is especially likely to occur if there is a history of ambivalence in the relationship.

Ambivalence may be particularly notable where there has been emotional conflict or *experienced* rejection or devaluation, (that is, even if there is not a conscious intention on the part of the other) as well as where there has been emotional, physical, or sexual abuse. When the subjective tension between attachment longing and feeling abandoned or violated increases, there may be heightened aggression that is simultaneously directed inward and outward. In the mourning process the negative side of the ambivalence (hurt and angry feelings, and blaming of self and other) may lead to

psychological and social disruptions, and the person is especially
in need of empathic understanding. Empathic attention to such
heightened ambivalence is particularly attentive to the emotional
violence directed toward the self.

HANK

I met Hank, who lived in a supported independent living situation, about three years after his father's death. He was referred for treatment because he had begun to break residential and workshop rules, to spend rent and food money impulsively, to act out sexually in self-destructive behaviors and to have fits of temper. These behaviors started just after his father's death, but subsided soon after. There had been a series of recurrences of this behavior. The recent outbreak of these impulsive, disruptive, and angry actions was more intense, and staff, after a team discussion about Hank's behaviors, thought that Hank's behavioral disturbances were expressing continued grief over his father's death, and referred him for an evaluation for grief therapy.

Hank's relationship with his father was a complicated, powerful, disturbing undercurrent throughout his life. His father, an alcoholic prone to fits of rage, was emotionally abusive to Hank. Hank's self-loathing was a legacy from his father, who violently cursed and insulted him. But, his father also spent close and very special time with Hank, sharing his love of the railroad with Hank. They rode the local commuter trains, and played with father's model trains. These continued to be Hank's favorite activities. Hank identified with his father, and was very connected to him. I asked Hank how he felt about his father. He said, "I hate my father and I love my father!"

A couple of months after the acting out that had precipitated treatment started, it stopped. This had been the pattern that had been occurring since his father's death. When he stopped acting out he felt ashamed of himself for his bad behavior, and he was anxious that he would be punished. Hank begged for reconciliation with his residential support staff, and urged that he be forgiven for "making a mistake." In the repentant aftermath of his acting out he was strongly engaged with staff and demonstrated a clear and confident sense of purpose. He was filled with the hope of reconciliation with staff, and was committed to make this happen. When we tried to understand

Hank's grief behavior we needed to look at both parts of the grief enactment, the destructive acting out and the reconciliation.

Hank behaviorally 1) acted out the inner turmoil of his grief, and then 2) sought forgiveness. He enacted a self-destructive drama, felt the disapproval of staff, felt guilt and abandonment, and then sought reconciliation. His ambivalent relationship with his father compelled him to repeatedly enact this guilt drama. He was deeply ashamed of himself for being so bad and destructive and out of control, and sought to repair the damage he had done. The drama was motivated by a persistent guilt and shame. Each time he went through the acting behavior and the seeking reconciliation behavior, he got staff disapproval and then staff acceptance. Afterward, he did well for a while, then repeated the pattern. Why did he not succeed in really achieving reconciliation?

I think that it is because the acting out was also an expression of anger at his father. His guilt was only half the problem. The other half remained unacknowledged. The response to his acting out was disapproval of his problem behavior. And he, in turn, responded to this by accepting responsibility and behaving as he was expected. He was able to do something *to try to repair the pain that was bound up with his ambivalence toward his father. He created this drama, in which he took responsibility for his anger, and there was peace for a while, but what he was angry about was bypassed. I think that because what he was angry about in the first place never got dealt with, conflict broke out again. The unrecognized part of the picture was that his acting out was an angry protest against his father's injurious behavior. In his ambivalence toward his father he was able to affirm his love for his father by doing what he was supposed to do, but what he was angry about was ignored: justice has not been done. His injuries and his anger about being hurt, which propelled the complicated grief behavior, had not been given its due. After protesting his father's abusive behavior toward him, he took the blame. Even though he was forgiven, in his underlying vulnerability, he was unfairly accused. It was his father who needed to be forgiven. The grief drama he enacted was the voice of his guilt, but his relationship with his father was not one in which he was the guilty party! His father was emotionally violent toward Hank. The whole drama of guilt and forgiveness invalidated his traumatic woundedness at his father's hands. It invalidated the claim he was trying to assert in his destructive rage against his father's psychological violence toward him.*

The bind of ambivalence for Hank was that in order for him to forgive himself for his hatred of his father he needed his father to take responsibility for his violence against him. But, dead or alive, his father was unable to give this to him.

AGGRESSION, ANGER, HATRED, REVENGE, INDIFFERENCE, PARANOIA, ETC.: DEATH AS AN ACCUSATION

Aggressive behavior is a distress signal. Increased compulsivity and increased aggression are two primary indicators of psychological distress among persons with mental retardation. Aggression is an expression and a signal of the intrapsychic experience of the violence of loss, a reflexive reaction to the implicit violence of loss. Aggression counters the utter helplessness and mortification of loss and gives back the pain that is experienced in the loss. Aggressive grief behavior is a language which expresses the inner distress of feeling that a loss is inflicting aggression directed against oneself, and is a common grief reaction in persons with mental retardation.

Some losses or some aspects of a loss are experienced as psychological violence that cannot be symbolized. An inner experience of being violently assaulted may be behaviorally expressed as aggression. The experience of being violated by a loss is, perhaps, what knocks a person into shock and numbness in their initial reaction. This sense of violence may persist in the recurrent realization of the loss, over the course of mourning, feelings of a rejection or abandonment which violate one's sense of security and self-worth.

As we saw above in the case of Hank, the supportive environments need to be especially careful not to take the disruptive behavior to be the problem, or fail to focus concern on the grief that is expressed by aggressive behavior. Aggressive behavior is a way of saying that something is wrong. The supportive task is to find out what is wrong and help the person deal with it.

BETTY

When I asked Betty about her mother's death, she said with uninhibited glee that she was glad her mother had died. I asked why. She said that her mother never gave her enough money, and added emphatically, "So I had to give up everything!" It is not clear what "give up everything" meant. Perhaps, it was the voice of her mother's frustration with and resentment toward Betty, that Betty repeats, signifying to herself over and over her mother's rejection. Or, perhaps, she wanted what her mother did not give her enough money to buy, more snacks, which signified to her the deprivation of what she felt most missing in her life, and blamed her mother for not giving her. While it was unclear what "give up everything" meant to her, I believed that it had to do with the pain in her relationship with her mother, and asked her if she had gotten enough love and affection from her mother. She said, tersely, that she loved her cat.

Saying that she did love her cat, in response to my question about feeling loved, seemed to say that she did not feel loved (by her mother), but that she was able to give love (to her cat), and felt gratification in being able to give love. The candid and startling pronouncement that she was glad her mother was dead was expressed in a voice filled with a vehement, hateful resentment and vengeance. She seemed consumed by a bitter wound of the deprivation she felt in her relationship with her mother. But she did love her cat, and this nurtured her woundedness, compensated for her being deprived of what she needed most, and abated some part of her resentment.

A further noteworthy behavior was that she compulsively begged for money to buy treats. This behavior seems to be expressing the same wound expressed in her grief over her mother's death, that is, feeling deprived of something she most desperately needed. The narcissistic spitefulness of her aggressive speech was a protest about having "to give up everything." Her aggressive language about her mother's death gave a highly condensed picture of an injury, "So I had to give up everything!," that appeared to shape and preoccupy so much of her emotional life. In her chronic grief others were not to be trusted, and could only be used to try to get money for snacks, begging and manipulating, as she did with her mother, to try to get back what she had lost: "everything."

CAROLINE

I met Caroline a few months after her mother's death. She told me she was very close to her mother and admired her deeply. Later, I learned that the relationship was also "very stormy." Staff said that since her mother's death "she has been getting upset often" and "has *been short tempered with housemates and staff" and striking out at everyone around her. She had become extremely sensitive to the mildest criticism, and sometimes when she felt criticized, her body became rigid and constricted. She alternated between distancing and clingy behaviors, which had been a pattern prior to her mother's death (suggesting insecurity and narcissistic volatility), but this had gotten much worse since her mother's death.*

Caroline told me that her mother died in the hospital, where she had been for more than a week before her death. At first, she could only say that she was angry and confused that her mother had died, and kept saying that she couldn't understand it. She said, "I can't believe it." This expression usually means "I can't believe she has died." But, it soon became clear that she also meant something else by this.

In response to questions about the death, Caroline said that no one told her that her mother was sick or dying. She did not learn of her mother's death until afterwards. Because her mother did not beckon her to her bedside to say goodbye, she felt like she did not matter. She was so shocked by the impact of the thought that her mother did not, after all, love her, that she became confused and filled with rage. She was not able to actually think the thought that occurred to her when she learned of her mother's death. The thought that tormented her was, "I can't believe that she really didn't care."

Caroline's verbal aggression toward her housemates and staff expressed her outrage. She reported several staff for treating her abusively. The staff were suspended and transferred. She told me that it was a lie. She said that she lied because she was so mad. The clever and vicious deed of taking out her revenge on whomever she could, expressed her sense of being betrayed and of the deep insult she experienced in her mother's death. She said that was "able to make staff leave." Perhaps, exercising the power to send away was an attempt to master the injury of her mother so rudely taking leave of her. She felt "abused" by her mother's abandoning her, and, acted out toward staff the revenge she wanted for her mother.

We talked a lot about her mother and her relationship with her mother. I pointed out that in attacking others she was really expressing how angry and hurt she was at her mother, and she easily made the link. We talked about her feelings of being left out, spurned, and abandoned by her mother's death. We talked about the history of this feeling as an undercurrent in her otherwise loving relationship with her mother. It turns out to have been a powerful trend in the relationship. Her mother had a very active social life, and traveled a lot, and Caroline was often left behind. And in this feeling of abandonment, she experienced herself as not really worthwhile nor loved, and blamed her mother for this. This injury was, in her mind, in some way, the same as the emotional injury she felt about having cerebral palsy. They both signified for her being left behind, unable to be like her mother. Being wounded and enraged by this, which had been in the background all her life as chronic mild depression, flared up intensely after her mother's death.

Meetings were arranged with her father and with her brother so that she could ask her father why she was left out, and for us together to talk to her brother about his telling her to "get over it and stop talking about mother." She refused to speak to her brother since he said that to her. Her father said that neither he nor her mother had anticipated the death. Mother was in the hospital and doing OK Unexpectedly, he was called late at night and told that she had just died. The next morning he called Caroline and told her of the death. She was not relieved at all by this explanation, and did not believe that he was telling her the truth. She merely felt excluded and devalued again because she believed he was lying to her. She said that he was just saying this to try to make her feel better. In her meeting with her brother the rift between them was repaired enough that she resumed talking to him, and felt much less angry at him.

We continued to talk about her relationship with her mother, and her feelings about having cerebral palsy. Her anger at her mother and at herself eased up some. A cemetery visit was arranged. Caroline chose to go with a staff support person, rather than a family member. Her acting out behaviors stopped. She continued to feel hurt and angry, but it was much milder and less disturbing. Gradually the focus of treatment shifted from her missing her mother, and feelings associated specifically with that, to her being angry that she had cerebral palsy, and could not do things which she wanted to do.

SARAH

Sarah had been sexually abused at a residential placement when she was twenty-two years old. Immediately after this she returned home, and continued to live at home. Her mother reported that Sarah was very upset at the time, but this was only for a brief period, and she did not appear to have been traumatized. I met her many years later when she was 40. It was just after her father's death and she had begun to have episodes of violent verbal attacks toward her mother.

When her father died, Sarah lost the security and confidence of feeling valued by him. Her mother was very devoted and caring, but got easily frustrated with Sarah, and did not make her feel good about herself. An underlying wound of worthlessness anxiety which her father's presence had mitigated against, was now threatening her, and was associated with her relationship with her mother. Her grief over her father's death was expressed in her raging at her mother, and a heightened anxiety about her self-worth.

The factors that contributed to this narcissistic vulnerability were the absence of her father's reassuring presence, an underlying ambivalence in her relationship with her mother, and the traumatizing violation of the sexual abuse. Her complex grief reaction of verbal aggression against her mother was, in one sense, a delayed reaction to the sexual abuse, triggered by the loss of her father's protective presence. The violation she experienced in the sexual abuse damaged her sense of self-worth, her sense of satisfaction with herself, and her underlying sense of security.

After her father's death, whenever her mother expressed disapproval for any behavior, Sarah took it as an insult and an attack. She attacked back with raging insults and screams at her mother, that reflected just how violent the injury was that she herself was experiencing. After a time, she began initiating verbal assaults from out of the blue, indicating that thoughts and feelings of being insulted and humiliated by her mother were habitually on her mind. She was severely depressed.

After visiting an office building, Sarah came home raging, and said that she saw women who had money, nice clothes and briefcases, and why didn't she. Her rage expressed her feeling that her mother hated her and was responsible for her narcissistic wound of not being good enough. We see here how the traumatic injury years prior to her father's death came out after his death as harsh, intense feelings of devaluation which she experienced as coming from her mother, in whom she experienced herself as not good enough.

JIMMY

Jimmy had been demonstrating significantly increased aggressive behavior. He had a characterological tendency to exhibit *aggression when frustrated, but had recently been more aggressive, and had thrown a chair in his workshop. A staff person at the workshop on whom Jimmy had a big crush had recently gotten married, and Jimmy felt jilted. Jimmy took her marriage as a devastating loss. He had invested his sense of manliness, an important part of his identity, in believing that she was his girlfriend. I asked him how he felt about her marriage. He said, with a wide dismissive sweep of his hand, with a very much in control and tough guy tone in his voice, that it was "Nooo problem!" This expressed both his defensive denial of the big problem he didn't want to face, but also the confidence he felt in feeling control over the problem at the time we were talking. It may also have been a promise or an oath he was making to me.*

In any case, he was frightened of his vulnerability and he covered it over with an exaggerated macho attitude. His grief over his experienced rejection and loss of a love bond involved a narcissistic regression to severe temper tantrums which expressed feelings of arrogance and grandiosity. For Jimmy this was a normal grief reaction, but it was a disturbance for his social environment, and communicated that he was experiencing a painful disturbance. His rueful, intimidating gestures were narcissistic defenses, protests against a loss of self, against feeling helpless, worthless, powerless, and small. Jimmy could not acknowledge his injury without being overwhelmed by the shame of it, which, no doubt, triggered his blinding rage. Yet, as he calmed down from the intensity of injury and rage, many months after the loss occurred, he was able to talk about the loss with resignation and disappointment, and with no aggression nor regressed affect.

When, during a grief therapy session, Jimmy enacted an aggressive scene—shouting and gesturing that he was going to throw a chair, I stood directly in front of him, and firmly told him to put the chair down, that it was not permitted. Then, I said to him that I thought he went around trying to intimidate people whenever he felt a little threatened himself. I emphasized his intimidating intentions, and how much pleasure he got from pushing people around that way. I told him that he liked to act like such a tough guy, and like nobody was going to push him around, because he knew how to push other people around, and he was good at it—but he was going to have to cut it out. He could not go around trying to intimidate and threaten people. For the first time since I'd known him, about three months, he made direct eye contact with me. Then he smiled, laughed heartily, and said, "You're smart! You're real smart." He may have meant that I was a wise guy like him. Or, he may have just been taken aback by the confrontation, and put it this way because he equated being smart with having power. He was smart, too, in getting control of the situation back, by manipulating me with praise.

But, I was glad for his approval, and he started to treat me with more respect. He was reciprocating the respect I showed him by talking with him man to man, and calling him on his behavior without blame or rancor. He may have appreciated the control when he was himself probably frightened of getting out of control. I think that his treating me with more respect was most of all a reciprocation, and an expression of our mutuality. At the moment that he said, "You're smart! You're real smart!," a very particular sense of bondedness, filled with mutual admiration, occurred between us. He reached out and shook my hand, smiled at me in a gesture that expressed recognition. I said to him, "You're smart!" He looked at me with wise guy, cocky satisfaction.

Whenever Jimmy started to feel out of control, he panicked, and tried to take control of the situation with aggressive, threatening, and attacking behavior. He threatened, intimidated, and verbally abused people, as a way of trying to regulate an acutely sensitive, paranoid vulnerability to feeling made "small" and powerless. His mother tended to baby him, and he lived with an undertow anxiety that she was trying to control him. His aggression, in this light, expressed a desire for autonomy, and seemed, most of all, to be a protest against powerlessness. Grief aggressions in persons with mental retardation may, in a basic way, be a reaction to underlying helplessness anxiety.

SOMATIZATION

Somatization is the psychological process of converting psychological pain into physical pain or into a physical disorder. For example, chronic stomach pain may be a somatization of grief. In the treatment of such a somatic disorder the therapeutic aim is usually to help the person experience the pain that is avoided by the somatization. In this defensive process, the body becomes an expressive instrument of grief. The therapeutic strategy in such cases is usually to identify the feelings and make links to the somatic symptoms, so that the psychological pain can be experienced.

In the case that follows treatment developed in a different way, based upon the initiative taken by the client, Milo, to use treatment to heal himself. This case in unusual in many ways, as the reader will soon realize. The case presentation here is longer than other cases because of the richness and unusual nature of the clinical material. The way the material unfolds in this recounting is based upon the unique way in which Milo presented himself in treatment.

MILO

This is a case of an unusual use of symbolic thought processes and magical thinking to provide security against grief that had, initially, been somatized into intense, chronic stomach pain. Through the use of symbolic enactments of the omnipotence of his cognitions, the client was able to confront his death anxiety, partially relinquish his omnipotent constructs, and reconcile with both his father's death and with his father. Milo, with an IQ of 43, was a brilliant performance artist. He had no deficit in his self-consciousness, his symbolic creativity, or his wit. Milo said of himself, "Some people think I'm stupid. I'm not that way to me. I'm clever and cute to me." The very unusual story that I tell here is an attempt to give a faithful account of a remarkable and very unusual man and his grief.

Milo, a young man with Down's syndrome, had stomach aches that were so painful and persistent that his mother sought extensive medical treatment. When all physical causes for his pain had been pursued and ruled out, she considered the possibility that Milo's stomach pains may have been an expression of grief over the deaths of both his father and his grandmother.

Milo's performance on the Wechsler Intelligence Scale for Children–Revised conducted about ten years before I met him yielded a Full Scale IQ of approximately 43. A psychologist who had seen him about five years before I met him reported that Milo "experienced difficulty expressing his thoughts and frequently struggles to communicate his ideas and opinions."

Milo, immediately upon sitting down in my consulting room, sprang back to his feet, and with raised voice and waving hands he gestured his mother out, and told me that he would talk to me privately. He said we would bring her in at the end of each session and that I would give her a summary of what we had talked about. My job was to listen and to write down what happened in the session.

I told Milo that his mother had brought him to see me because she thought that his stomach pains may have to do with feelings about his father's death, or his grandmother's death. I told him that she hoped I would be able to help him with his stomach pains and his grief.

He listened intently to what I said, and responded in a startling way. Immediately, and with great dramatic flair he announced himself to be Superman. He said he was the one who would stop death.

> *I'm going to stop this silly old game of death. It's up to me to stop it.*

From the moment he announced himself to be Superman, his stomach pain ceased.

Over the next year Milo created a fantastic story of his heroic defeat of death. He took complete control of our meetings, and his self-healing enactments only needed me to bear witness to his heroic deeds. He was very pleased with his thinking and self-expression, and did not seem to care much that others didn't recognize how very smart he was. He announced that there was

> *only one way to stop my death,*

and that was by the heroic performance, in poetic language and dramatic gesture, of his conquering death. Here is a beautiful example of his performance art. One day Milo came to see me dressed in jeans, a sweatshirt, and an outdoorsman's insulated vest. We had only just started the session when he began to make emphatic gestures that he was about to show me something of great importance. He then dramatically ripped open his snapped-up vest, and revealed a large Superman insignia in the middle of his sweatshirt. He beamed with immense satisfaction.

> *Look who I really am. I am Superman. You thought I was only kidding. Now you see it is real.*

He performed a symbolic realization. He pretended to fly around the room, and flexed his muscles to show his power. He was demonstrating this before me, and my seeing it and believing it was a necessary part of its effective power for him.

His mother, he said, depended upon him to stop death.

> *I want to stop my mom from dying. My mom went through a lot. But this time it's going to be my way around. . . . If someone pulls another death on me, I'll stop it. . . . I can be a dangerous man, a stranger to myself, being bad to help my parents.*

He threatened murderous death with his own murderous powers.

Milo oversaw the report he directed me make at the end of each session. He required that I end each session by reading my note for the day, and that I begin each session by reading to him what he had said in the previous session. I believe this was to make sure I got it right and to support the continuity from session to session.

Milo secured the symbolic sacred space of treatment as a space for his performance of symbolic reality, and protected it from being exposed as nothing but a lie. At the beginning of treatment Milo invited his mother in at the end of each session, and I read aloud my report on what Milo had said. A few weeks into the treatment Milo's mother said that Milo had a vivid and remarkable imagination and that he made things up. Milo disapproved of her saying this and forbade her from coming into the room again at the end of a session. He said she

> makes me have lies,

and

> I don't want my mom involved in my death, telling me lies.

Milo called the symbolic constructs by which he realized his defeat of death real. He secured the space in which he enacted the symbolic realization of his triumph over death by excluding the critical perspective that said this was merely playacting, and not real. He frequently expressed and dismissed concerns that he was "just kidding," or "that he was just "pretending," and that his magical performances and declarations were not true and real. In the context of the symbolic space in which he defeated death, what was most real was his power, his identity as Superman.

> I am Superman. Mom is not Superman. It's by me to stop it [death]. Serious . . . Do something about it. Will do it my way. I'm the one with the strength to stop it. Kauffman means Kauffman. But I'm the one to stop it. My name is called real.

Milo summoned the courage to overcome his helplessness and terror in the face of death, and, by saying his "name is 'real'," he asserted and magically laid claim to his identification with his symbolic consciousness as Superman who defeats death. The reality of his pronouncements and performances, resembling mythic reality, was established by his symbolic enactments.

Milo physically expressed how very powerful and brave he was not only with his words but with his gestures, and his voice and his *body language filled with bravado and signifying power. He gathered up a great sense of authority and bossiness and commanded that death will not ever happen again.*

> "My Mother [Milo called his maternal grandmother 'Mother,' the name his mother called her] was not strong enough," he said, with a gesture to show how strong he was.

> Being cute and clever, being silly? No! If someone is in danger, I have strength . . . Superman in me, for real. Pretending is one thing . . . I am super. It's the one way to stop death. It's me. I'm number one. And number two. I have to do something about it. Super means to stop my death again. By me.

A theme that ran through Milo's treatment was his belief that doctors had killed his father. His father died in the hospital, and Milo had seen medical staff hooking up an IV, and conducting other medical procedures. He experienced death as an act of violence, which had a paranoid element to it, but believing the doctors killed his father also gave him a concrete enemy to confront. The belief that doctors had killed his father existed in a way that was dissociated from his actual relationships with doctors. But the belief persisted, and in the following statement we see that toward the end of treatment, when he was able to partially acknowledge his fear and helplessness before death, he continued in his belief that the doctors had killed his father.

> Doctors scare me. They killed my parents . . . my own . . . I'm not that strong . . . in my Clark Kent suit I'm not strong.

Milo asserted acute awareness of "his self" as existing and subjectively present. He used emphatic speech, such as, "I was scared, myself scared,"—where the word myself *was used to emphasize his sense of himself as being scared. This was a way of pointing to his own self as fearful, of saying not just that he was scared, but that he was especially conscious of experiencing himself to be scared. He frequently used such emphatic expressions as a way of saying "my very own self," or "me-ness." He sometimes referred to this as being "personal." These expressions suggest a very well developed sense of himself. Milo also used the emphatic speech in another way that was similar to this, but instead of indicating his own identity, indicated the quintessential core of an idea. He said,*

> Strength is to have love. Love itself. Love. My mom and me.

In both ways of using emphatic speech I understood him to be signifying how full and vivid his sense of the world was.

Milo was keenly aware of the possibility of others dying and kept vigilant attention to the mortality of his loved ones.

Other people are getting death all the time. I hate that. Even my own parents. Even my own father. Even my own mother.

He was prepared for another death and lived in an awareness that it could happen at any time.

Someone might try to pull another death on me. Again! Quickly!!

He lived on the alert. Alarmed by death, secured by his omnipotent symbolic productions and performances, he maintained a vigil in face of death.

Milo's father was a proud and highly respected prominent community, who, especially toward the end of his life, was prone to fits of rage and drunken, out of control, angry verbal assaults directed at Milo, Milo's mother and sister. This caused all of them great distress. Milo reports that

I told him to cut out the silly thing.

Milo had been angry at his father at the time of his father's death. He was most angry for the distress his father caused his mother and his sister and for the verbal violence directed at himself. Protesting against his father's violence, wanting to stop his father's alcoholism and raging assaults on the family, blurred into his anger at death, as, in both instances he invoked his omnipotent powers to put a stop to the violence. He expressed a complex mixture of hurt, anger, disappointment, sympathy, sadness, and other feelings toward his father.

One day, Milo, after a lot of painful discussion of his father, sang a prayer for him. He composed it on the spot. He closed his eyes and sang, very tenderly:

I miss you, Dad
I know, Dad, all the things you sent to me were not pleasant.

You shouldn't do things like that.
In death I miss you. I miss you.

He then cried "I miss my father, I miss my father!"

On occasion Milo spoke of God. His suggestive and clever language often radiated with insightful intelligence, and a creative awareness of himself and the power of his cognitions.

God is power. Like the lamp, it can go on or off. That's God.

This statement about God exemplifies his understanding of his own creative power, the light by which his symbolic world appears to him, the power of his cognition.

Milo talked about his sense of the contingency of his symbolic world, and the contingency of the power of his being Superman. I think the "going off" of the light is implicitly connected to the death that the powers which construct his symbolic world guard against; in his account of the power of God, death is present as concern about the power of his cognition being interrupted. His cognitions were deployed with the intent of defeating death. The power that he was most concerned with in his meetings with me was the super power of his own thinking. And, I was very struck by his describing power here as something that goes on and off, by his thought that the power of God goes off.

In a primary way, psychologically, he alluded here to his own vulnerability to death. I think that some such sense of his contingency is the meaning of his comment on God, and that in the foreground he lives in this power. God, in the foreground, was the power of the symbolic flying he engages in during our sessions, and in the back-ground was his mortality. While some readers may find it incredible that Milo could have expressed such complexity or subtlety of thought, I have no doubt that he understood what he was saying perfectly well, and in a very immediate and beautiful manner.

One day Milo and I had an interesting discussion about the power with which he stops death. He said,

My super thinking stops my death . . . will stop it before someone else dies . . . quickly.

By "quickly" he certainly meant "faster than death," otherwise it wouldn't be fast enough. He demonstrated this super thinking by performing a metaphor for "faster that a speeding bullet" or, as it were, "faster than time," by stretching out his arms in front of himself, gesturing that he was Superman flying.

I asked him what he was doing.

> He said, "it makes you fly."
> "How?," I asked
> "The wind gives you power."

I asked him to explain to me how this worked. He said that the wind was hidden inside his clothes.

> "You can't see it," he said. "The wind is power hidden inside me. . . ."

The wind was a metaphor for the power of his thinking. By this power, he beat death to the punch. When Milo said "super thinking," he was talking about a particular cognitive process that he experienced and identified with. When he talked about the wind being hidden, he was most emphatic about it being invisible. I think that once he started to talk about Superman flying he recognized the wind as a metaphor for the power of his thought and imagination. There was an expression on his face of particular pleasure in the thought of the hiddenness of the wind, and it seemed an apt metaphor for the creative power of his thinking.

He was, however, sometimes so enthralled by the hallucinogenic power of his super thinking that his consciousness was overwhelmed.

> Sometimes a storm is really powerful. Your brain is not even there. . . . Sometimes it makes you fly, yourself. . . . I feel great, but not when I think of my father. He was a tired old man. . . . He started all that stuff on Millie [his sister], and me and mom. I don't care about him anymore . . . I can deal with it when he starts yelling at me. . . .

The symbolic enactment of his power over death seemed to have helped him to overcome his fear of his father's violence. I say "seemed to," because it was not perfectly clear to me what happened in Milo's symbolic constructions that allowed his vulnerability to be tolerable and his self-confidence in dealing with his father to emerge. His fear of death, we may notice, was closely connected to his fear of his father.

> Sometimes I laugh in my head, but anymore sadness means to be happy again,

he said to me. Sometimes he spoke in a language that was opaque and suggestive, and this comment about "sadness means to be happy" may be such an expression. It is possible that he really meant to *say that he was no longer sad. I think, however, that he meant he was safe and secure enough to be able to feel his sadness. Connection to oneself and grounding in one's ability to live resigned to loss, and in integrating loss and sadness into oneself, even if transient, is not usually called happiness. Yet when Milo put it this way, I thought that he was expressing a fine outcome of mourning, and a very wise and beautiful understanding of happiness.*

SELF-LOATHING, SELF-DIRECTED ANGER, GUILT, SHAME, AND OTHER ATTACKS OF THE SELF

One of the most disturbing ways that grief expresses itself among persons with mental retardation is in the self-blame and aggression against oneself that occur in reaction to a loss. In nearly every case in this chapter on psychological complications there is an element of turning against oneself.

Turning against oneself includes guilt, sometimes virulent forms of guilt with very aggressive and compulsive attacks on oneself, as well as shame, including shame-based guilt and self-loathing. This reaction sometimes appears to be a primary reflexive action in response to loss. The self-blaming, self-destructive urge may link up with particular circumstances for which the grieving person blames him or herself, such as in the case of the person who said "I made her die with my problems," but there is, no less, an underlying tendency toward self-blame in the reactions of many persons to loss.

Criticizing oneself may involve severe frustration with oneself, self-hatred, self-annihilating rage, or wreaking havoc upon oneself. Turning against oneself may take the form, as in the case of Mark, below, of compulsively repeating, and, finally, craving the very humiliation that hounds and horrifies him. Turning against oneself tends toward an addictive-like psychodynamics of being compelled toward what one wants most to avoid, in a self-destructive course that seeks relief from the pain of loss: this is the psychodynamic of the *compulsivity* of turning against oneself. The compulsivity of this depressive state is that it seeks satisfaction and self-healing in self-destructive tendencies.

The self turning against itself in grief, with blaming and shaming attacks, is actually a classic psychoanalytic understanding of depression as an avoidance of the pain of grief. Turning against oneself was understood to be a reaction to loss, in which the grief stricken person turned against him or herself *instead* of mourning. We now recognize that this is a "normal" trend in mourning, which, however, may become a self-consuming preoccupation complicating mourning. Among persons with mental retardation there appears to be an increased vulnerability toward becoming preoccupied with attacking oneself with blame and shame.

In some instances of the self turning against itself in grief, persecutory anxieties are particularly evident. The self, attacking itself, experiences the attack as coming from other people; in attacking oneself the person experiences himself to be passive, and experiences the attack as coming from others. Relationships with others may be habitually experienced from the vulnerable position of feeling blamed and shamed by others. More primitive persecutory anxieties involve a poor differentiation between self and other, and attacks are experienced with an aggression in which self and other are undifferentiated. Attempts to strike out covertly turn back against oneself in blame and shame.

MARK

Mark had been doing quite well and was moved to a higher level of independent living. In the new residence his housemate was friendly and Mark quickly grew fond of him and attached to him. The new housemate, however, soon began to curse and insult Mark, telling him that he couldn't do anything.

Mark has cerebral palsy and walked with leg braces and crutches. His new housemate told him that he couldn't walk. Soon Mark's walking grew worse. He began to lose confidence in himself. He obsessed over not being able to walk and could soon no longer walk. He started to fall. He was given a walker, and even still could barely ambulate.

Mark began to feel anxious about getting to the bathroom on time, and out of this anxiety he started urinating in his pants. He felt incompetent and was humiliated by wetting himself. As his abilities deteriorated he became more and more frustrated with himself, and his situation continued to worsen. He obsessed and despaired over the hopelessness of his situation, and grew more and more angry with himself and ashamed.

Mark's pattern of deteriorating behavior is a disturbing language of self-annihilation; he got caught up in a magical, self-fulfilling, obsessional downward spiral of behaviors that enacted escalating self-defeat. He felt helpless, despairing and full of self-loathing, and in an effort to overcome the treachery of this, in a perverse effort to regain control, he further lost control, as he began, in the middle of the night, to pile his clothes on the floor of his bedroom, and to urinate on the pile. He told me in a manner that said he couldn't believe that he did this, expressing disbelief and embarrassment.

The whole manner of his telling me about this conveyed not only defeat and humiliation, but a vague hint of satisfaction, a faint giddiness about it. I asked him if he had gotten any pleasure out of peeing on his clothes. He responded with a slow building, then uncontrollable, sense of glee. Urinating on his clothes on the floor in the middle of the night was triumph over the humiliation of peeing in his pants, in which he felt himself to be out of control and reliving the humiliation of his not being able to walk, a pervasive shame of "not being able." His glee was a celebration of victory over humiliation by an act in which he simultaneously succumbed *to humiliation and* chose *to humiliate himself, an act of self-annihilation in face of* helplessly *dying of embarrassment, shame, and defilement.*

His wish to achieve mastery over the helplessness of the loss experience fused with a self-destructive impulse which the loss experience triggered. He attempted to find pleasure and mastery by deliberately inflicting a loss of control upon himself, rather than being subjected to it, yet, there was, at the same time, guilt and self-punishment in his repetition of the loss. His submission to the self annihilating significance of a loss was an act of self-sacrifice to appease his rage and disappointment.

Talking to me, he was at first baffled and surprised at his own behavior, and had no idea of what he was doing, as if the manic celebration of his humiliation had occurred in a dissociated state of which he was just now becoming aware. In a strange triumph over the loss-of-control and humiliation, he created a secret ritual of self-humiliation. We see here how turning against oneself in humiliation can escalate, as anxiety about loss of control fosters 1) increased loss of control and 2) a compulsion to humiliate oneself in a final act of succumbing to the insult of "not being able." The line between subjection and mastery disintegrates, and Mark made not being able to walk and get to the bathroom on time into a self-destructive, heroic, secret ritual of being able (to pee on his clothes in a pile in the middle of his bedroom floor in the middle of the night). For Mark this was an ultimate relief from his shame.

PHILLIP

Phillip had an obsession about holding his mother's hand. Eventually, when he was 44 years old, his mother's annoyance peaked and she told him that his hand holding had become a nuisance. She and Phillip's father had also believed that Phillip was indulging romantic fantasies when holding his mother's hand, and were severely disapproving of this. Phillip said that when he was holding her hand he thought about old happy memories of being with people he liked and of pleasant experiences he had with his mother. He also expressed feelings of physical affection for his mother. He said that he liked holding his mother's hand more than anything else.

When he was forbidden from holding her hand, he reacted by destroying his most valued possession, his music collection. He repeated, as his grief reaction, the experience of loss that had just been inflicted upon him. Perhaps his music tapes and the meaning of listening to music were associated with his mother, but it was, no less, his habit, when experiencing a loss, to attack himself by destroying something he valued.

One of the most perplexing and remarkable grief reactions, which is typically associated with traumatic loss, but is not limited to it, is re-enactment of the loss experience. This is understood by ego psychology as an effort by the ego to master the loss, particularly the helplessness at the traumatic core of the loss. This concept is a useful and meaningful way to understand this self-destructive trend in grief, but there is more to the disturbing repetition of the loss than this view accounts for. There is not only an element of self-hatred and self-blame in the re-enactments, but there is primitive reflex of the self turning against itself in grief in human nature, which is particularly evident in some persons with mental retardation.

Phillip's self-rage was temporarily appeased by the act of destroying his tape collection; but it did not resolve the injury, and he continued to dwell within the loss, repeating self-destructive behaviors from time to time as an expression of his undying claim on his mother's hand, and his deeply seething grief. He struggled for a couple of years with bitter resentment and was not able to accept her decision, or redirect his desire.

Then, during a phone call with his mother on the day before the 4th of July, Phillip told his mother he changed his mind about coming to visit for the holiday weekend. Afterwards, in a session in which he was far more talkative and lucid than usual, he began the session by telling me that he had made a decision. He said his mother called him and his sister guests in her house, and he did not want to be a guest in his parent's home. He decided that he was going to become more independent, do more things for himself, as staff had been encouraging him to do, and he decided that he no longer wanted to hold her hand. He said he was annoyed with how his parents were treating him, and he didn't know why he had to wait so long to learn this. He blamed his parents for allowing his dependency to go on so long, and all he wanted now was to learn to do more things on his own. The issue was not yet settled, but his stepping outside the dependency position he'd been stuck in with his mother, significantly reduced his self-destructive behavior.

MANNY

Manny's compulsive hand biting had developed when he was young, first in reaction to his father's anger at him, expressing, I think, anger at his father, and frustration with himself for being "bad." He had been a very curious child and took apart everything he got his hands on in order to try to figure out how it worked, destroying valuable property, like his father's accordion. Sometimes, such as when he attempted to dismantle the furnace, his behavior was dangerous. As he learned to restrain himself from doing certain things, he cultivated an intense and furious anger with himself, and an enduring guilt and shame having to do with the internalized storm of his father's rage. Hand-biting was a language in which he expressed his frustration and anger at himself.

As an adult Manny was chronically at risk of responding to nearly every frustration with a hand biting attack, and sometimes, like Phillip, intentionally destroying his own most valued possessions, such as his treasured photographs of an actress which he cooed over and caressed as a way of comforting himself.

After an episode of self-directed violence he felt pity for himself and comforted himself by looking at pictures of women, eating food, and cuddling with objects (such as socks, bananas, and a male housemate whom he said reminded him of his mother). So far as I can tell, his mother had taken pity on him, and comforted him by holding him after his father's verbal attacks.

Treatment was aimed at helping him develop less harsh self-judgments and a less self-pitying sense of comfort in his internal life. We talked abut the frustration and anger he felt with himself, which was expressed by his hand biting. I tried to help him to find peace and reconciliation with his angry father, who continued to live in him. We addressed his being so frustrated and angry with himself for so long, and sometimes talked about his self-anger as his father being angry at him. In treatment I encouraged him to forgive and make peace with his father and with himself.

He developed a small degree of self-regulation, and was able to restrain himself, and not bite himself, some of the time. Manny learned to be able to calm himself better after hand-biting episodes, by "taking relaxation," which was putting his head down on a table, or lying down in bed. We talked about this as a way to let go of the bad feelings, and fill up with good feelings about himself. Hand biting continued to be his language for anger at himself, but, very gradually, it became less intense and less frequent. He began to sometimes merely put his hand to his mouth and growl at himself, gesturing hand biting, without actually biting.

JASON

The much loved administrator at the workshop where Jason was employed died, and I was asked to conduct a bereavement group for those most affected by his death. I went around with a staff person meeting and gathering together the persons who were to be in the group. When we approached Jason I was introduced, and told him why I was there. I said that the administrator had died, and before I could say another word he started shouting that he hadn't done it! In the group he repeated this vehement phrase several times. A couple of years later when I was back again at the same agency conducting a bereavement group after the death of a worker, I met Jason again. We went around the table, each person talking about the person who'd died. When I came to Jason he said, "I didn't do it!" He repeated this a number of times, and that was all he said.

Jason's tone that conveyed to me a feeling that he was lying, that is, that he didn't believe that he didn't do it. His denial seemed to express a feeling that he really was guilty. He repeated the denial in a very rigid, ritualistic, obsessional, urgent, and unconvincing way. He was not very successfully defending against self-annihilating guilt, demonstrating both a rigid preoccupation with persecutory anxieties, and a defensive structure in which he did not have a lot of confidence.

Jason's paranoia reflected a pervasive and primitive anxiety that he would be blamed. He was chronically and deeply preoccupied with an anxiety that he had done something terribly wrong, and he experienced many situations as accusations. So threatening was this anxiety that he was prevented from experiencing any other signification in the loss. All he could experience was a total blaming assault that threatened to annihilate him. The compelling and overwhelming power of being at fault for something he couldn't comprehend precluded all other possibilities of experience for him, and prevented him from mourning. All he could do was try to mount a defense against the accusation by saying "I didn't do it!" His primitive, obsessional guilt and paranoia limited his awareness of himself and the world severely. Much of his psychological existence seemed to be consumed by this preoccupation. This condition, which, in Jason, is severe, may be present in varying degrees in other persons.

CHRONIC LOW LEVEL ANXIETY AS NARCISSISTIC GRIEF

Some persons with mental retardation live with a chronic sense of self-dissatisfaction and self-criticism. The self-attacks may not have the intensity, big gestures or drama we've seen in other grief behaviors described here but are present as chronic low level narcissistic anxiety, or chronic grief over a loss of self-esteem. These may periodically flare up in response to diverse stressors registering as narcissistic injuries, or occur as anxiety reactions in interpersonal interactions, in facing change, or in task performance situations. This is usually diagnosed as depression. It is a type of grief many persons experience, though the depth, chronicity and the influence on functioning of this type of depression varies from person to person. We have seen it as a factor in several cases discussed here, and it is particularly evident in "higher functioning" persons with mental retardation, who have a disturbing awareness of not being able to do things other persons can do, such as not being able to drive a car, not being able to have a baby and family, or in not having other symbols of social "normalcy." In the case that follows it is more a matter of a feeling of self-consciousness, and not fitting in with her peers that reflects a chronic loss-of-self anxiety.

DONNA

Donna was a 38-year-old woman who lived at home with her mother and father. Her mother brought her to see me because she was withdrawing from social activities with her friends and she reported that this behavior had occurred off and on over the years.

When her mother was present in the session Donna was inhibited; when asked questions, she demurred, pouted, looked embarrassed, and turned away. She brushed aside her mother's worries, both annoyed and indulgent. But, when her mother left the room, she came alive with excitement, and talked non-stop.

The self-consciousness she expressed in her mother's presence was similar to what she felt in socially isolating herself. She felt objectified and embarrassed, which is a condition that may be called "exposure anxiety."

Donna was a fanatic lover of sports. She and her father watched and talked about sports together and she had strong opinions and a command of details about baseball, football, and ice hockey. Each session Donna dazzled me with details about the games that occurred the previous week. She had a fine, cynical sense of humor about sports, which she got from her father. The story line when she talked about sports was always what players had done wrong, and what they should have done. She worked washing dishes, and was knowledge-able about every aspect of operations in the kitchen. The stories she told about the kitchen had the same feel—she talked about mistakes people made, including herself, with stern and annoyed disapproval (in the manner of her supervisor, I gather). She knew her job well, and was proud of her ability, but occasionally made mistakes, from which she was able to learn and reaffirm herself. In social situations, however, where she felt exposure anxiety and narcissistic vulner-ability, and where there was not the structure that existed at work, but, rather, open ended interaction with peers, she was fearful that she would do something wrong, feel ashamed and rejected, and, in anticipation of this, was self-conscious and nervous. Why this had recently become much worse for her was not clear, but I suspect there had been some interaction with her friends in which she had felt their disapproval.

When I asked Donna about her worries and her frustrations with things going wrong, she looked thoughtful and sad, and sat still and silent for a long time. Then, she said that she felt frustrated over a lot of things. In response to my questions, she said that she had felt frustrated for a long time, for as long as she could remember, since she was a little girl. She said she had never talked about it before, but it was always there. (And, after this one occasion, she never spoke about it again.) She said that she was frustrated when she didn't do things right. She was chronically anxious that she would do something wrong, and would feel ashamed of herself.

At work, Donna's embarrassment over doing things wrong could be resolved through learning from the experience and doing things right. This enhanced her self-esteem, and self-confidence. Her employment was a part of her life where she strengthened her sense of self-confidence a lot. And her pleasure in and knowledge about sports, also strengthened her positive self-regard. But a low grade narcissistic anxiety continued to disrupt her life, particularly in social relations, and her social withdrawal expressed anxiety of not being good enough, as having done something wrong. In the shame about being seen by others as not good enough, she felt separated from others and rejected, and withdrew in abandonment anxiety and a loss of self-worth. The only behavioral expression of this pervasive, but often well managed feeling, was her social withdrawal.

Since her parents were in their late 70s, Donna, her parents, and I worked out a plan for Donna to move into a supported independent living environment while they were still able to support her with the adjustment process. But each time things were settled and the placement plan began to go forward Donna changed her mind. It was here, in the context of dealing with this change from living at home to living in an apartment (in a big apartment building where several floors were rented by persons with mental retardation), that I found an effective approach for addressing the chronic narcissistic anxiety expressed in her social withdrawal behavior.

Donna's anxiety about the change did not have to do so much with leaving the safety and familiarity of her parents' home as with the feeling that she would not know how to do things on her own, and especially that she would not know how to fit in with the others at a new residence, and that she would feel left out. Her adjustment process to the new residence, with coordinated support from her parents, myself, and especially agency staff, was helpful in reducing the level of chronic narcissistic anxiety felt in social situations (often called social anxiety). She was, in this new social environment, able to become a bit more comfortable with herself in peer socialization.

THOUGHTS ON THE RELATION OF COMPLICATIONS IN THE GRIEF OF PERSONS WITH MENTAL RETARDATION TO PSYCHODYNAMICS OF GRIEF IN ALL PERSONS

It seems to me that the expressive language of persons with mental retardation brings to light aspects of the grief of human beings generally that have not been clearly recognized in our cultural self-understanding of grief, nor articulated in our theories of grief. Aspects of grief explored above, particularly, 1) *aggression* directed outward, as well as self-loathing, shame, and other aggressions against oneself, and 2) *compulsivity* are important aspects of grief in all persons, though not as behaviorally evident as in the expressive language of grief in persons with mental retardation.

Aggression toward self and others and compulsive tendencies are basic psychodynamic forces and normal undercurrents of grief in all people that appear to me to be especially revealing about the nature of human grief, but not clearly recognized by the constructs which organize our understanding of grief and mourning.

Aggression and compulsivity are two basic modes of reaction to loss, and increases in aggression toward self or others, or increases in aggressivity or compulsivity are presumptive indicators of grief distress. Among persons with mental retardation we often see aggression and compulsivity enacted in global, physical, and direct ways. In persons without mental retardation these trends are less global, physical, and unmediated, but, I think, just as basic as reactions to the disruption of psychological order perpetrated by change and other loss, including death.

If we try to identify the core of grief by looking at the acute experience of grief in the initial reaction to loss, we may be able to recognize a traumatic shock which registers an experience of violence to the self. The self can only respond to this shock with global denial or a dissociation of the reality of the loss. In persons with mental retardation this primitive, intense breech of the self's integrity, safety, and everyday orderliness tends to be responded to with increases in expressions of compulsivity and aggressivity.

In others, that is, persons without mental retardation, aggression often has a more complex social overlay, in which the disturbances are manifest in interpersonal conflict, disillusionment and dissonance, narcissistic depression riddled with defenses, and complex, sometimes subtle patterns of turning against oneself; and, occasionally, there may be situations of more physical and direct expressions of anger and aggression.

In all persons, including person with mental retardation, compulsivity functions to conserve the status quo, to prevent change, and in the service of an urge to restore lost assumptions by continuing to believe, in diverse ways, that what is gone is not gone, what has changed has not changed. Compulsivity functions defensively in grief to help maintain a sense of constancy. Perhaps in persons with mental retardation there is a greater vulnerability to the flux in which humans exist, a weaker barrier against the inward thrust of mortality, so that aggression and compulsivity are more pronounced as a reaction to this imposing presence of death and its threat of annihilation.

CHAPTER 5

Program Development: The Creation of a Grief Supportive Community
•
Guidelines for Agencies

INTRODUCTION: PREPARATION FOR RESPONDING TO LOSSES

Agencies may become grief supportive communities by developing a range of programs that will support client loss issues. This chapter describes a number of basic programs that an agency may develop, but the set of topics covered here is intended give a set of examples of programs that many agencies may wish to adopt, and is not intended to be comprehensive.

Program development has two general goals:

1. To establish procedures, services, policies, and protocols that care for the loss and mourning needs in a community in which persons with mental retardation live, and for these to be developed into standard practices and standards of practice;
2. To raise awareness and understanding of the meaning and impact of losses, and the healing that may be achieved in mourning. To raise levels of knowledge and competence among staff in being able to support the mourning of the persons they work with.

Agency program development is a concern not only of agencies, but is also a concern of grief counselors and therapists who may help agencies develop grief support services as a part of the clinical intervention aimed at helping the supportive environment in which the person lives to support the grief needs of the person.

The agencies that are primarily considered in this chapter are residential service agencies. Other types of agencies will find some of the program initiatives discussed in this chapter useful, and are encouraged to become familiar with grief issues and grief support programming ideas, so that grief support needs are understood and integrated into agency services, as suitable. Also, residential agencies may wish to have a staff person who has training in grief counseling, who can coordinate the development and implementation of agency grief support programs.

Handling death in the life of an agency, and in the lives of persons with mental retardation is a matter for most thoughtful concern in an agency's self-understanding as a supportive environment. The way the experience of a death of a family member, for example, is supported will influence the inner life and expressive behavior of the client in the deepest most enduring ways. When a death (or other significant loss) impacts the life of a client, it reverberates powerfully in the heart, and his or her psychological existence.

This is a matter for attentive and intentional concern, expressed in interpersonal supportive relationships, in agency practices and agency policies. Agency standards of practice which respect the human dignity and vulnerability of persons with mental retardation, and which are the expression of compassionate love through agency policies and practices must be especially attentive to the experience and expression of loss in people's lives.

AGENCY LOSS TEAM

The function of the *Agency Loss Team* is to be aware of and take care of the loss and mourning needs of the agency. An agency may approach the task of developing an *Agency Loss Team,* by opening up a discussion of loss experiences and perceived needs, and out of this expression of concern and discussion, invite persons to be part of a team. This is most likely to take place in the wake of a loss that raises staff awareness about the importance of being able to support persons when losses occur. At such a time recognition of the need for knowledge and protocols is likely to have momentum. But it certainly need not be in reaction to a particular loss situation that a decision is taken to develop an *Agency Loss Team.*

The team consists of a cross section of agency staff. A person with mental retardation should be on the team, and involvement of a family member on the team should be considered. Persons who are interested, who are in a position to make things happen in the agency, and who are representative of different perspectives within the agency may also be considered.

A first task of the team will be to assess agency needs, and develop a set of priorities for program development; there is likely to be a lot that the team will want to do, and it will take time to develop a full range of grief support programming, so the team will have to decide its priorities.

The assessment process that is carried out by the *Agency Loss Team* should seek input from the entire agency—all staff (including management), clients (whenever possible), and families (if feasible) should be invited to share concerns and perceptions. Broad-based participation in the assessment process gets wider input and involvement, helps to generate awareness, and assures that many in the "community" have a voice and a stake in the process.

The team develops programs for the agency, such as training programs and protocols for responding to losses, and is *involved* in responding to losses by supporting staff most directly involved and coordinating services for persons who are grieving. The assessment process enables the *Agency Loss Team* to identify loss-related issues that need policy and program development. Setting up these policies and programs enables the agency to be prepared for losses as they occur in the life of the agency. It is always useful to build into the process periodic self-evaluation by the team in order to adjust policies and programs to better meet needs.

The *Agency Loss Team* is the hub of the agency's preparedness to respond to and support losses in the life of the agency. Interventions are directed to the client to help facilitate the mourning process, and to staff and families, in order to help staff and families support clients. As a part of getting its bearings, *Agency Loss Team* members may wish to discuss, as a group, losses that each member has experienced. This can be a powerful experience, and everyone on the team should feel safe, and no one should feel any obligation to talk about their own losses. The team may want to have this discussion facilitated by an outside facilitator.

The team has to assess: 1) grief and loss needs of individuals, groups of individuals, and the agency as a whole that are presently active, based upon an assessment of losses that persons have experienced or upon behaviors that persons exhibit; and 2) program development initiatives that are needed, a part of which should address specific situations that have occurred in the life of the agency. This guidebook is a tool that the team may use to help in identifying and designing responses to grief support needs, and to develop an agency handbook of policies and practices for supporting grief and mourning needs within the agency.

When a loss occurs the team meets with the staff most directly involved to develop a support plan and to provide support to these persons. The team supports by listening to the concerns of the direct care staff and by giving: 1) guidance and direction; 2) specific and concrete support interventions; and 3) validation to the staff. Listening to the observations and feelings of staff is an important part of the team's response to a loss in the agency. The team also provides direct support to the grieving person by talking to him or her about the loss, and engaging the person in ways that provide: 1) support to the grieving person, and 2) assessment information to the team. This meeting may take place once, occasionally, or more regularly, based upon the team's decision about the needs of the person. Out of this assessment with staff and the grieving person or persons, the team comes up with a support plan that may include ways staff can support the person in day to day interactions, activities or rituals needed, extra support or therapeutic intervention, etc.

There are many program development directions in which an *Agency Loss Team* may go, and many different concerns it may choose to address. The team may be more effective if it does not simply try to follow a formula, but in considering the suggestions advanced here, to think creatively about their own situation. Teams may develop a great variety of concerns and interests over time.

Here are sample minutes from a meeting of an actual agency support team meeting:

Grief/Loss Committee Meeting Minutes. April 7, 1998

We seem to be on track with the information discussed at our last meeting.

1. The loss assessment [see topic *client loss assessment* in this chapter, below]. We added some possibilities as to what it might look like and/or information that should be included. In addition to previously decided information we felt it might be best for the house advocate to complete prior to the yearly plan and that it would be reviewed at each meeting. In more critical situations it could be completed sooner. We each had ideas what it would look like in completed form. We decided each of us would complete a trial with one individual. We will review at our next meeting to compile information and create a finished product.

2. Staff exit interview [see topic *staff turnover and other broken relationships* in this chapter, below]. Questions we would like added to the exit interview were reviewed. It will be listed in the employee handbook that upon termination these questions will be addressed.

3. The memorial. The proposal will be addressed to Steve. We read plans for the development of a memorial. Barbara will look for a universal statement plaque. We thought that a beautiful place with a gazebo would be developed. Each month something new could be added, e.g., a plant, a bird feeder, a flower box, etc. We will need to have a path to the gazebo. Pictures will be included in the gazebo.

4. Training [see topic *staff training* in this chapter, below]. The training scheduled for April 22 will be taped. We will discuss further training programs at future committee meetings.

5. Is there a need to have regular times for people to come together to share grief related memories? This could be added to the training. Dedicate the last half hour or hour to training specifically for that purpose.

6. Next meeting will be May 20th from 1:30 to 3. Remember to bring your completed assessments.

AGENCY SELF-ASSESSMENT OF LOSS EXPERIENCES

Agencies and sites within an agency have a history of losses that are part of the life history of the agency. The emotional life of a community living arrangement (CLA), a workshop, other facility or of a family does not exist in a historical vacuum, but is part of a continuum of experiences over time. Losses that have happened in the past are as much a part of the life of an agency, as are past losses a part of the life of an individual. The impact and the meaning of these historical events may significantly affect the psychological environment of individuals living or working in that environment.

When an agency has been through a loss the response of the agency to the loss is also a part of the legacy. Persons affected by the loss may come together in a supportive and healing way, and the experience may enhance the sense of security, strengthen the sense of self and the supportive efficacy of the environment. However, the reverse is also true. The loss experience may have a disruptive effect and injuries are etched into the life, expectations and self-experience of individuals and agencies. In general, these two trends may each occur to some extent in every loss event. Whatever way an agency grief process is played out in reaction to a given loss will have some bearing on subsequent loss experiences.

Assessing agency loss experiences is a process that helps develop some perspective on the agency as a psychosocial whole, as well as on individual loss experiences of persons served, whose grief is experienced in the context of social environment of the agency. The general questions are "what losses have affected the lives of persons in the agency?," "what have been the agency supportive responses?," and "what has been the course of grief in individuals and, to the extent that it applies, in the agency as a whole?"

The *Agency Loss Team* may want to find ways of setting up the agency loss assessment process agency-wide, with units or sites within the agency conducting their own grief self-assessments. The self-assessment process may then function as part of an agency-wide educational agenda.

Such an assessment may also function as a tool in the psychological preparation of an agency for the process of developing loss support services, and might sometimes be helpful to do again at other times, as staff changes, as an ongoing self-assessment, or as other circumstances may indicate. The self-assessment process is, in a way, an implicit mourning process, as the loss team or the agency as a whole talks about agency grief experiences, how losses were handled, and continuing grief concerns.

Life is deepened and matured by mourning. To the extent that losses are avoided or the mourning process becomes otherwise stuck, development that is possible through mourning will not happen. If the humanizing that occurs in mourning is blocked, there is a risk that a vacancy or disconnect may open in the heart of human bondedness in an agency. In its responses to mourning the character of an agency's caring may mature.

When an agency evaluates the history of it's own loss experiences, the inherent healing possibilities of an agency grief support program are nurtured. Agency loss self-assessment prepares the way for grief support program development.

The Agency Self-Assessment Process

The task of this assessment is to identify past losses, and the responses and consequences of these experiences. Discuss and make a list of answers to the following questions:

1. What losses have affected the agency as a whole, a specific site or an individual?
2. How, *at the time the loss occurred* had individuals been affected?
3. How had the staff and the agency as a whole responded to the loss?
4. How has the loss continued to affect feelings and thoughts and be part of how present situations are experienced? How is it being dealt with now?
5. How do you plan to deal now with continuing consequences of the loss?
6. How would you deal with similar situations in the future?

A self-assessment process may be designed and implemented by the *Agency Loss Team.* An outside facilitator may be used to help the team accomplish this. The consultant may conduct grief trainings, facilitate the team's process of designing and implementing the agency self-assessment, or otherwise helps the team get started with agency grief support services.

CLIENT LOSS ASSESSMENT

The loss assessment aims to put into words: 1) the story of the losses a person has experienced, 2) the reactions, and in particular the disturbances that have occurred in reaction to these losses, and 3) the course of the adaptive process.

A client loss assessment is an important part of the intake process for new clients. The history should include deaths, other broken relationships, and other losses that have occurred in the life of the client (including, and especially, the placement or change that is occurring at intake), disappointments, separation, other difficult changes, as well as the person's reactions to these losses. Behavioral changes and ways that frustrations are responded to should be carefully noted, and the relation of these to loss events should be considered. When an agency first implements a policy of intake loss assessments as a part of the standard assessment process, a plan should be developed for conducting a loss assessment with current clients.

The purposes of the initial loss evaluation may include:

1. gathering information;
2. opening up discussion of loss and death topics may be beneficial in simply the act of having losses recognized, and in being given a meaningful opportunity to talk about losses; implicit in this is the expression of concern, and permission to talk about losses, that is, sanctioning mourning;
3. building relationships with family and client, as the discussion of losses may help to strengthen the bond of trust and mutuality;
4. educational opportunity regarding relationship issues, loss issues, death issues may occur in the course of the assessment;
5. talking about losses in assessment interviews may help the mourning process; this is particularly so with regard to the changes that are occurring, of which the intake is a part, the crisis and adjustment process of placement, or adjustments to transfer, or new employment; since the agency will be immediately supporting the person through mourning and adjusting to this change, this is a key area for the agency to have an understanding of, and a preliminary support plan;
6. developing a written instrument that can be used in ongoing evaluation process, tracking changes and helping staff to make links between behaviors and experiences over the course of time;
7. setting the scene for decision-making processes, such as setting up advance directives;
8. heightening awareness of loss and mourning; and
9. developing a document that will be used by direct care staff in understanding psychosocial needs and in providing a picture of the grief vulnerabilities and behaviors of a client.

SUPPORTING STAFF AS A WAY OF
CULTIVATING AN AGENCY
CLIMATE OF GRIEF SUPPORT

The interpersonal relationship between persons with mental retardation and staff may be a very important dimension of the grief experience of the person with mental retardation. Assuring and maintaining staff equanimity in reaction to losses requires careful attention by management to staff needs for support with job frustrations. Staff frustrations may come out when under the stress of responding to client's grief behaviors. Creating and managing an agency climate that is safe and able to provide caring support in response to sometimes disruptive grief behaviors is an important concern of management. The relationship between staff and the person with mental retardation is a vital part of the emotional environment in which the person experiences the pain of loss and the hope of healing. And a role of management is supporting these relationships.

The losses clients experience affect staff, and sometimes staff can be helped in understanding their own reactions, or trained in supportive responses to grief that do not make the person feel wrong or bad for his or her grief behavior. Staff's own feelings of fear, frustration, or insecurity may incite non-supportive responses to a client's grief behaviors, such as controlling or reprimanding/blaming the grieving person.

Underlying any agency policy for dealing with losses are basic attitudes that affect supportive responses to the expression of grief's pain. The attitude of management toward staff may affect the attitude of staff toward clients. In developing attitudes that will best support the mourning needs of clients, it is important that staff's own feelings and experiences of loss be considered, and staff be supported in being able to respond with concern and compassion to disturbing and disruptive grief behaviors.

Six aspects of developing healthy staff grief support attitudes are:

1. provide support to staff in dealing with loss situations, attending to the loss experience of clients' *and* staff's own loss experience, including discussions of difficult grief behaviors of clients or providing a facilitated group to support staff processing difficult client grief behaviors;

2. provide training for staff to help staff to (a) understand client grief needs and expressive grief behaviors, and (b) use their relationship with clients to support and facilitate the mourning process;
3. listen and be responsive to staff needs, concerns and frustrations in handling client grief issues;
4. develop effective bi-directional communication, up and down the supervisory chain of command communication about client loss experiences and behaviors;
5. nurture and exemplify concern with the quality of caring relationships in which grief may be expressed;
6. help staff maintain a professional and respectful perspective in dealing with client's grief behaviors and affects.

These six dimensions focus on the care of the relationship network, the agency's human environment in which clients experience themselves, relate to others, and are supported in dealing with the disturbances of grief. The most important ingredient in the services provided to a client experiencing a loss is the compassion that is there in the helping relationship.

To establish a caring community for clients to live in requires establishing a caring community for staff to work in. What this means in terms of agency structures is the development of a structure in which staff losses are listened to and supported. The creation of a safe and supportive atmosphere for staff is critical in building a nurturing agency atmosphere for clients. Attitudes ground practices and policies for dealing with loss and mourning. Careful attention to staff attitudes is pivotal in assuring that the programs that are developed will be meaningfully integrated into the lived experience of clients' relationship with staff.

STAFF TURNOVER

Staff turnover is a pervasive and sometimes insidious loss experience for clients. Clients need to form meaningful relationships with persons in their support environment. If these relationships are impoverished, the human environment in which the client lives is likely to be damaged. The emotional meaning of the interactions between staff and client in the course of the routines of the helping relationship is an important part of the clients emotional life and mourning process. Staff-client relationships are both:

1. a primary source of nurturance of the human bond, and
2. the *human context* in which other support tasks are carried out.

Staff turnover presents clients with broken relationships again and again. Repeated loss tends to undermine the ability to attach. It becomes too risky, and the quality of attachments may be compromised. A person is less likely to feel safe to open up to a new relationship, when the wounds of the loss of the previous relationships counsel one against it. When experience has taught that new relationships will lead to abandonment and rejection, a wall is built up to limit exposure to an otherwise longed for attachment. The frustrated need for deeper connection tends to be played out as damaged self-esteem and/or interpersonal conflict. The need for connection is, for most persons, fundamental for well being.

If we cannot eliminate staff turnover, nor prevent the wounds of loss that it tends to inflict, we can develop approaches to manage the staff turnover process in a way that will care for the wounds it inflicts. And sometimes when a staff person is leaving it can be a healing and nurturing experience. The aim is to manage the breaking of the relationship in a way that maximizes the client's adaptive responses.

In order for us to get a perspective on the termination process in the helping relationship, I will try to put termination in the context of the whole relationship. The phase-process model of helping relationships looks at the helping relationship over time in terms of a beginning phase, a middle phase, and a termination phase. We will take a moment to consider each of these phases, so that we may see how the termination phase (which is, psychologically, a separation experience) is integral throughout the life history of the staff-client relationship, and in order to understand termination as a process in which needs key to a person's experience of grief are addressed.

The Beginning Phase of the Helping Relationship

When new staff begin their training an important part of the supervisory process is focused on:

1. the significance of their relationship with clients;

2. the transience of the relationship, i.e., that it has a beginning, a middle, and an end, and what this means in the client's experience and in their own experience;
3. the history and impact of other staff relationships in the life of the clients with whom the new staff person will be working; this includes past and present staff relationships, and in particular the termination-separation process with the staff person they are replacing;
4. the assessment of losses and broken relationships in the life of the client, including a review of the loss and broken relationship intake assessment—losses experienced, how the loss was responded to by the grieving person and by the supportive environment at the time it happened, and continuing consequences of the loss experience in the life of the client; this and #3 provide information *and* cultivate empathy;
5. beginning the ongoing attention that will be paid in the supervisory process to developing and using the relationship with the client to support the client;
6. the skills and attitudes for managing and using the helping relationship with the client in ways that will best serve the client's well being, including our concern here with the person's grief;
7. the importance and value of the staff person's dealing with his or her own feelings in her relationship with the client.

In the supervisory process the supervisor may model the professional supportive and nurturing attitude.

The Middle Phase of the Helping Relationship

The middle part of the relationship involves relationship building and the management and use of the relationship in helping the client. Among the many important issues that are present in the relationship are the ways that the client brings his or her loss experiences into the relationship. Residual and underlying chronic feelings of loss, that is, unresolved grief issues, are likely to be enacted in the helping relationship, and this establishes an interpersonal context in which grief issues are processed over the course of the relationship.

The Termination Phase of the Helping Relationship

The termination phase of the relationship is the intentional process of achieving as meaningful as possible a closure to the helping relationship. We have discussed the beginning and middle phases here, partially in order to clarify and focus the termination phase in the context of the whole helping relationship. The overview of a phase-process model of the helping relationship illuminates the meaningfulness of the care that the termination phase of the helping relationship calls for. Saying goodbye, and the whole way that the end is negotiated, carries an enduring message about the relationship— and what that relationship says about oneself and one's own life, place in the world, value, lovability, etc.

To say goodbye is to seal a relationship, i.e., goodbyes are sometimes experienced as a time when the measure of the relationship is taken ("Do I really matter to this person or not?"). Many persons are especially sensitive to separations because of vulnerability to the experience of abandonment, and negation of one's worth. Termination may be a tender and vulnerable time in a helping relationship.

It may be helpful in several ways if staff understands the meaning of the termination process from the beginning of their job. The staff person should, whenever possible, give sufficient notice so that the process of working through the ending of the helping relationship may be thoughtfully carried out. The amount of time needed for this process will vary, with three to four weeks being typical. Staff are sometimes able to and interested in keeping periodic contact with the client after termination of the helping relationship. In most instances this may be supported. It gives an opportunity to affirm and validate a special relationship after termination, and may provide the context for further working through of issues in the relationship. It may express a genuine sense of friendship and caring that survives the end of the helping relationship.

The termination process is carried out simultaneously in the relationship between:

1. the staff person and the client,
2. the staff person and the supervisor, and
3. the staff person with other staff.

The goals of the termination process are:

1. to validate and affirm the value of the relationship;

2. to deal honestly with conflicts and differences and do as much as possible to help the client find resolution to problems or tensions in the relationship, and to acknowledge the client's strengths;
3. to share the staff person's own feelings about the relationship and the loss of relationship with client;
4. to help the client deal with the separation and loss;
5. for staff to express gratitude for being able to serve, help, and get to know the client;
6. to say goodbye.

It may be helpful as part of the termination process for the departing staff person to spend some special time with each person he or she has a significant relationship with. The period of time during which the relationship is intentionally focused on the task of saying goodbye is treated as a special time in the helping relationship.

In some instances the client may personalize termination. The loss of the relationship may mean abandonment, loss of security, guilt ("I did something that made you leave" "you are punishing me by leaving"), shame ("I'm not good enough for you to want to stay"); it may link up with other losses (other staff leaving, death of a parent or placement, or residue from any other loss experiences); or it may, as already noted, link up with stresses or conflicts in the relationship.

In the supervisory process at termination the supervisor helps the staff person:

1. decide on the timing and approach to the client in announcing that he or she is leaving;
2. assess the issues that need to be addressed with the client in the termination process;
3. assess his or her own feelings about leaving, the work that needs to be done with the supervisor, and with the client to achieve a meaningful closure;
4. help the staff person support the client's separation;
5. respond in the most helpful ways to the issues that come up in the termination process with the client.

The supervision process during termination is focused on helping the staff person grow as they are working at saying goodbye; helping the staff person assess the successes and difficulties of the relationship with the client and decide on goals for the termination process; helping staff talk about the meaningfulness of their work and acknowledge their own satisfactions and disappointments; and to affirm and support the terminating staff person's accomplishments.

When a staff person is fired the planned termination process usually cannot be followed. If it is feasible for the departing staff person to have a face to face goodbye with clients, this should be done, even if it is necessary for this to happen with a supervisor present. In any case, clients deserve the respect of a goodbye and some account of the reason for leaving. If the departure involves disturbing issues for a client, provide the opportunity to talk through these issues.

STAFF TRAINING PROGRAMS

Staff training is an integral part of program development. It is a good starting place for agency program development. Staff training in loss and grief centers on the following concerns:

1. concepts and knowledge about grief, loss, relationships, broken relationships, aging, illness, death and related concepts;
2. talk about these topics being implicitly and explicitly sanctioned, and for discussions of these topics to occur among staff in the training;
3. staff to have the opportunity to talk and share among each other experiences of loss and death in their own lives;
4. staff to look at client behaviors they have dealt with and recognize the grief and the mourning needs expressed in these behaviors;
5. learning skills, strategies, and approaches for supporting clients dealing with losses;
6. introducing agency programs, policies and procedures for dealing with loss, or discussion of needs for policies and procedures, as a step toward further program development;
7. staff and agency as a whole to increasing awareness, understanding, openness, and sensitivity to loss and grief issues;
8. the agency using the training as a step toward establishing norms and standards practice for dealing with losses;
9. staff being engaged in thinking about client losses, services needed to respond to specific client losses;

10. staff beginning to develop a competence and a confidence in responding to client loss languages and needs; and
11. staff being stimulated to learn more.

As the reader can tell from this list, grief and loss training may be customized for the needs and wishes of the particular agency, and this may be worked out in preliminary consultations between the trainer and the agency. Some agencies will want just a brief introduction to grief and loss, a two or three hour training program and others will want more extensive training programs. So the trainer, in collaboration with the agency, may need to decide what topics are most pertinent to the needs of the agency. Often for brief programs I use the same outline, but cover material in less depth or limit the amount of time for group discussion. The staff training may be stretched out over long periods of time, with different segments at different times, or shaped to meet evolving needs. The training may be taped or digitally recorded, and shown to others, though the obvious disadvantage of this is that those watching the playback cannot participate. New trainings may be conducted as the agency learns more through experience in applying learning from previous trainings, or to respond to staff turnover. Training may also be a response to a particular loss that has occurred, focused on issues germane to that situation, and combined, with a supportive inter-vention, such as a grief processing group, or consultation on handling a particular issue. Administrators, senior managers, and supervisors, as well as direct care staff, should be encouraged to participate in the agency grief training program. The down side of this, which may weigh against including managers and supervisors is if the presence of these persons would inhibit group discussion.

I have often found it to be helpful for staff to discuss loss and mourning issues of clients past and present, and for staff to feel welcome and safe to share losses in their own lives. This engages staff in the learning on a level which is most likely to be meaningful and useful. Furthermore, loss and mourning and especially death is a highly emotionally charged subject, and so a pivotal part of the training involves dealing with one's own responses in a safe and honest way.

The training program may, as indicated above, be used to initiate staff involvement in developing grief support programs, policies, and procedures. It may be the opportunity to announce an agency loss assessment process, to introduce or to recruit for the *Agency Loss*

Team, to seek input in developing new program initiatives, or to announce new program initiatives the *Agency Loss Team* is planning.

The training should be developed and carried out in a way which is sensitive to the particular concerns of the agency. What follows is a sample outline for a training program.

1. A General Introduction to the Mourning Process

The content of this section of the curriculum is the same as would be presented at a general introductory training program on loss and mourning. Every trainer will have his or her own approach to presenting basic topics and concerns and helping participants understand grief and loss. Here is an example of general introductory topics that I have used:

a. the meaning of loss and mourning in human life;
b. the inevitability of loss and death in human experience;
c. the deep spiritual and emotional significance of caring concern for the injuries of loss and death; grief is a universal human experience that cuts to the very deepest part of our soul and is the vulnerable core of our identity;
d. losses in normal development, such as the separation-individuation process, and throughout the life-cycle;
e. the phenomenology of the mourning process. There are many theories and the trainer may present a number of different theoretical schemes for conceptualizing grief and mourning;
f. the power of denial and the urge to avoid affects and thoughts of the loss; adaptive and maladaptive aspects of denial; the need for the griever to realize and experience the impact of a loss, to experience whatever pain is there; this should include attention to the need for staff to recognize and being open to pain; social tendencies to encourage denial; the value of social support;
g. the range of "normal" mourning; the normalcy of overwhelming psychological distress/disturbance in mourning; problems with the concept of normalcy;
h. disenfranchised grief; anniversary reactions; and other special topics; and
i. complicated mourning; risk factors for complicated mourning.

2. The Special Characteristics of the Mourning
   Process with Person with Mental Retardation

Chapter 3, "The language of grief," and Chapter 4, "Psychological concerns and complications" in this guidebook lay out the special characteristics of grief in persons with mental retardation, which may be used in approaching this topic. The training agenda for this topic can: 1) address the basic similarity of the grief of a person with mental retardation and other people, 2) focus the behavioral expressive language of grief in persons with mental retardation, and 3) describe the particular tendencies noted in Chapter 4, such as compulsivity, somatization, aggression, etc. The vulnerability of persons with mental retardation to narcissistic injury, the intensity of grief expression, and other topics to help staff develop a more deeply empathic understanding of the expressions of grief in persons with retardation, can also be included in the agenda. In this regard the trainer can help staff recognize that disturbing behaviors are not to be faulted or mistaken as bad behavior in any way, but understood as expressions of pain and grief. The trainer also may want to help staff appreciate the often open-ended time frames of the grief process.

In this part of the agenda, having participants present situations they have worked with or are working with would be especially useful.

3. How to Help Clients with Their Grief

The basic helping functions are to support and facilitate the mourning process, and to support adjustment to change. There are many examples in this guidebook of ways agency staff may help persons with mental retardation mourn and adapt to change, especially in Chapter 2, "Support Guidelines." The following is a sample list of topics that a trainer may use to get started in teaching staff to support the client and facilitate the mourning process:

a. help persons to talk about loss experiences, and empower persons to express grief;
b. work at understanding what the person's affective and behavioral grief language is expressing;
c. respond intentionally and validate affective and behavioral grief language and other expressions of grief;

 d. provide other supportive and grief counseling interventions, as needed;

 e. use the supportive relationship to help the client;

 f. be patient and prepared to work with the person's grief for an extended period of time;

 g. use teamwork and communication among staff;

 h. use rituals in helping clients with losses;

 i. involve families to help when indicated;

 j. use a support group as tool for working with grief, when several persons are affected by a loss;

 k. develop interventions that provide concrete experiences aimed at facilitating the mourning process, e.g., visiting the cemetery, making a memory book, visiting memory-significant places, creating a memorial place or memorial event, etc.

4. Other Losses

Other losses that may be addressed in the staff training program on grief include:

 a. losses related to staff employment termination;

 b. losses related to narcissistic injury, such as damaged self concepts or self-esteem, feelings of deprivation, feelings of abandonment, etc. (as discussed, for example, in Chapter 4); and

 c. losses related to broken relationships, especially family relationships and staff relationships (this may include material on the importance of these relationships in the lives of persons with mental retardation).

5. Case Discussions

This section may be integrated into other parts of the training. In this outline, case discussions may be particularly apt in Parts 2 and 3. Here I want to provide a few comments on using case discussions that are introduced by participants. An introduction to talking about cases may include some comments on the helping relationship, on supporting the dignity and maximizing the autonomy of the person with mental retardation, on the psychological and spiritual meaning of the helping relationship, or in validating the difficulty of some situations.

In case discussions the trainer focuses on understanding grief behavior, supporting staff in handling difficulties and frustrations they may have in responding to a person's grief behavior, and in developing an intervention plan for supporting the grieving person.

Sometimes staff may feel distress over not being able to "take away" the painful feeling or disturbing behavior associated with grief, and may need help in understanding that "taking away" the pain is not the goal of grief support. In cases of very disturbing or persistent expressions of grief, staff may need help in accepting and living with this pain, in maintaining hope and confidence, and in not trying to control the person's expressions of grief. Case discussions may be opportunities for staff to process their feelings and reactions to the case. The trainer may also encourage mutual input and support among staff.

6. Agency Structures, Policies and Procedures for Dealing with Loss and Mourning Issues

The agency may choose to use some part of the training program to address agency needs for program development, and involve staff who are participating in the training in this process.

7. Self-Awareness of Staff's Own Loss and Mourning Issues

A theme that is in the background throughout the training, for each participant, is one's own mortality, and vulnerability to losses. Sometimes in the course of the training this theme comes into the foreground, usually in regard to grief that a participant has experienced in his or her life. It is often helpful for the trainer to mention at the beginning of a training that one's own issues may come up, and to normalize this and give permission to participants to express and talk about their own issues, to the extent that will be possible in the time frame allotted.

In an implicit way, participants' awareness of their own mortality and grief is the touchstone of understanding the grief of the persons they work with. The trainer should be attuned to this implicit significance of death and loss, and may wish to find ways of acknowledging and addressing this explicitly.

PLACEMENT: CRISIS AND PROCESS

The Crisis of Placement

Placement in a residential setting should be done with careful planning for minimizing disruption and facilitating adjustment. We have already talked about how disruptive *change* may be for a person with mental retardation. Residential placement, especially when it is done at the time a primary caregiver has died, is likely to be the most difficult change in a person's life, and there is a significant risk of long term psychological complications as a result.

Residential placement is a major life crisis. The residential agency can make a great difference in the psychological health of the person by following admissions procedures that are thoughtfully and carefully attentive to the psychological vulnerabilities of the person, and maximizing opportunities for adjustment. Even when there is a transfer from another agency or location, that is, not an initial placement, the psychosocial meaning and impact needs to be carefully assessed and taken into account in planning the transition so as to minimize complications.

When a person with mental retardation is placed outside the home they lose the security of a familiar world that they so much depend upon. The loss of home is loss of the physical world, routines, one's very sense of identity and security. Home is both a part of self and self itself. It is where one experiences oneself and knows oneself. Home is the status quo of the concrete world in which one exists, the maternal nest, the safe place! Home is the place of the teacups and towels that one is attached to as the visual and embodied reality of one's very own sense of existence. Home is where family connectedness exists, and is where the person feels a sense of belonging.

The symbolic meaning of placement is, for many, abandonment. Being torn from the security and concrete bondedness of the physical environment can be devastating. The loss of home is often a traumatic loss; attachment to the human environment and to the whole world of familiar, known, predictable reality is endangered.

While there is, in the act of placement, a naturally occurring sense of abandonment and rejection, some persons have been told by a frustrated primary caregiver, "I'll put you away," or a similar punishment-abandonment threat. It is common to internalize this in negative self-concepts, guilt and the like. Even if the threat is not explicit, many persons feel it. Then, when a placement occurs, the psychological meaning of placement is that the threat has become a reality, intensifying and complicating feelings of guilt and abandonment that might otherwise be occurring.

The pain, insult and wound which the placement may inflict may persist for an indefinite period of time as an undercurrent, even after the person achieves a satisfactory adjustment to the new environment (which often occurs over a 9 to 12 month period).

MEG

Meg's story articulates the pain of abandonment anxiety. Meg was a 46-year-old woman who described her feelings about her residential placement (it had occurred many years prior to our meeting): "If anyone cared, he wouldn't put me in a car and just drive away. I want to be home. He made me feel like a criminal. I was very sad, depressed. My weight got too thin." She had been anorexic. "I am paranoid," she said. In response to my asking her what the word paranoid meant, she said, "Paranoid means I can't fight back. They might hurt me."

In this sensitive, gentle, and insightful young woman, a sense of abandonment in which she is helpless and emotionally assaulted is the prominent feature of her grief, and a troubling undertow in her everyday sense of herself. This woman had no "behavior problems." She had a depressed mood, but did not socially isolate, lash out at others, develop somatic symptoms, or exhibit increased compulsivity. She was very unhappy and hurt by her experience of abandonment, but was not symptomatic. Even though she demonstrated the egological resources to function in the world asymptomatically, she no less needed support to help her with the pain and inward emotional aggression of the abandonment of placement.

The Placement Process, as a Policy of Residential Agencies

The placement process, as a support policy of residential agencies, is the process the agency intentionally carries out for the purpose of helping the client mourn losses and adapt to the new environment.

Whenever possible gradual accommodation to help the person become familiar with the new environment should be provided. The agency should, whenever this is applicable, help the primary caregiver and the family to support the placement process by helping them engage the person in the process, providing interpersonal security and support, maximizing opportunities for familiarization, etc., as did the family of Marla (discussed in Chapter 2, in the section called "Support the adaptation needs of the grieving person"). Planning ahead may help to prepare the person, in whatever ways possible, for the new and unfamiliar environment, and secure memories of the lost environment. Policy may aim to empower through providing real choice or through other supportive interventions. The placement process should afford maximum client involvement.

When is the best time for a placement? This is a good question for families to begin asking before the issues become critical. There is a discussion of this in Chapter 2, in a section called "preparation for the death of a primary caretaker." A basic guiding principle is that when a person is prepared for a change, the adaptive process is supported.

When there is no planning ahead, or inadequate planning, and complications do occur in adjusting to the new environment, then providing opportunities to experience a connection to lost places and people may be useful; or goodbye rituals may be developed so the person can experience some connection to what is lost, and say goodbye. In conjunction with this, providing a welcoming sense of security and belonging to the newcomer, may be of great benefit. Patience may, in some cases, be required to support a person through a long, difficult adjustment process.

The actual day of placement is a special day, and gestures of welcome that treat the newcomer in a way that helps them feel at home and belonging and valued are in order. It may be a fun task for staff and other residents to think up great ways to welcome a new member to the CLA family. The process of saying goodbye to the previous resident and welcoming the new one may be a work of mourning and adjustment to change for all the residents at a facility.

The process of adjusting to placement occurs over a period of time; above, I suggested 9 to 12 months. This time frame may be typical, but should not necessarily be taken as normative. Whether the person has no turbulence at all, and adjusts right away, or whether placement is an open-ended process of reckoning with the loss of home, the supportive task is to recognize the grief that is there, validate the person, and help them handle the grief disturbances they express.

If the adjustment to the new environment is conceptualized as a series of stages, we might break it down this way:

1. feeling lost, displaced and disorganized;
2. trying to organize self to new situation and make sense out of new experience;
3. beginning to build relationships with other clients and staff;
4. developing a sense of belonging, connection and relationship.

While these stages are articulated here as discrete and sequential, like all schematizations of psychological process, it is never so neat or orderly.

This description of stages of adjustment is a part of a process of mourning the losses that are incurred at placement. Forming a new sense of belonging with other clients and staff at the CLA takes place simultaneously with grieving the loss of primary caregivers and home, and are two aspects, sometimes complexly interconnected, of the same process.

Sometimes the new client's reactions may not be evident. In some instances the grief reaction is delayed and emerges some time later (with no awareness that it is related to grief), as, for example, disturbances of mood, relationship, or behavior.

AGING AND ILLNESS

Agencies are more and more faced with issues of aging. And, as aging persons tend to develop chronic health problems, and, sometimes physically deteriorate, staff and fellow residents or workshop peers worry about the sick person and about sickness, and sometimes, about dying. Also, sudden illnesses and hospitalizations of a person at a site tend to arouse anxiety, and some degree of crisis for other persons at the site.

The primary task this sets for grief support is to manage the anxiety. The first problem staff tends to experience is their own anxiety and sense of helplessness. Staff needs a plan of action, a sense of knowing what to do, and supervisory support in managing their own anxiety and grief. These are achieved through communication and connectedness. When developing an agency plan to handle chronic or acute illness, the basic tasks are to communicate what is happening and how persons are feeling, and to nurture a sense of connection.

Information about the illness needs to be appropriately communicated to staff and to clients, and opportunities to ask questions about the facts need to be provided. Opportunities should also be provided for processing feelings, asking questions, clarifying misconceptions, and finding meaning.

Communication around a loss that an agency is experiencing involves:

1. sharing and clarifying the facts and practical implications of the situation;
2. processing persons' reactions over time, while the illness is occurring, both formally and informally;
3. sharing feelings, mutual support and experiencing the loss and anxiety as shared with others;
4. initiating a decision-making process, if feasible, to do something, such as visiting the hospital or sending a card (especially one made by the group) or a gift, or praying; and
5. finding meaning, for example, through stories that define and help contain the emotional experience of the situation.

A basic agency responsibility when there is an emotional crisis of any kind for a group of residents or workshop peers is to foster connectedness. The anxieties aroused in an emotional crisis may have many different sources, but loss of attachment anxiety is commonly a key aspect when an illness or similar loss is affecting a group. Even when anxiety involves subtle and complex disconnects from self and the social environment, it is likely to be helped by fostering a sense of connectedness. A basic aim or function of communication in an emotional crisis is to foster a sense of connectedness.

Such a process of agency self-care/client care helps to defuse and mitigate the grief complications that may be triggered in reaction to illness or other disturbances in the life of a residential or workshop group, and helps to assure security and safe passage through the difficult time. Care of communication and connectedness facilitates mourning and nurtures a sense of security in an agency dealing with client illness, death, or other group experience of loss anxieties.

In supporting persons who are faced with the illness or death of a peer or a staff person, there may, in some instances, be an appropriate occasion for client education.

CLIENT EDUCATION

Client education is an activity that is done, either when there is a loss that presents an occasion to teach something about death, loss, mourning, etc., or as an activity that is not in response to an event. The first of these is called a teachable moment.

Teachable moments provide good opportunities for educating clients about death, dying, and mourning. A teachable moment may be the death of an animal or plant, a death in the public arena that clients are aware of, deaths in the family of staff, etc. Lessons may be prepared before hand, and implemented when the occasion comes up.

There can be discussions: 1) about feelings, 2) about how people deal with different kinds of losses, 3) any grief related topics that staff thinks may be useful, or 4) open opportunities for persons to bring up their own concerns in relation to the loss issues that occasion the teaching session. Simply talking about an issue related to death and grief helps to normalize and to provide some context of cognitive and social meaning that supports dealing with death and grief. A primary function of these teachable moments is to prepare persons for dealing with grief experiences in their lives. Educational programming also may help persons develop a personal sense of the meaning of death and loss, and a degree of familiarity and comfort with a subject that is often forbidden and scary.

The moments in the life of an agency when a loss really impacts and needs to be grieved, and persons are grieving, are, in a psychosocial sense, teachable moments in which one *learns from experiences*. In this vein, the grief facilitation process may be understood from an educational perspective. Grief education occurs in actual client loss experiences. Education is implicit in memorial events or other rituals, in the day to day interactions between the grieving person and staff, in a grief processing group, in hospital visits, etc.

FAMILIES

My concern here is the relationship of families with residential clients, especially when family interactions with the person or with the agency are strained or when the person is experiencing abandonment. When families entirely or partially abandon a person, or whenever the needs of the person with mental retardation would be served by stronger family connection, it is within the purview of the agency to develop programming to support the person's need for greater family contact. This section is written in advocacy of the residential agency taking a stronger and more active role in helping to ameliorate the losses persons experience in feeling cut off from their families.

In approaching this it may be helpful for the residential agency to empathize with family members, and to find ways of helping them to feel more a part of the person's life. This involves reaching out to families in various ways. What is needed is for the person's "new family," the agency, to embrace the person's "original family." In order to be in a position to nurture the vital bond of persons to their families, the residential agency assumes an empathic and inclusive stance with families, especially with families of persons who are experiencing grief over the relationship with the family.

Family emotions in relation to the person may be complicated by guilt more than any other single factor. Guilt may be expressed by avoidance, controllingness, impatience, fostering dependency, criticism of staff and agency, or in other conflict-laden behaviors.

This behavior of a family member may be an expression of guilt over the feeling that he or she has failed and abandoned the person. The same behavior may also express ambivalence, i.e., the family member both loving and pushing away the client. As we attempt to put ourselves in the shoes of the family, especially alienating and alienated families, and can empathize with their pain we may begin to find ways to build bridges.

The role of residential facilities with families is both collaborative and educational. Collaborative means that the agency acts on the premise that family and agency are a partnership, each with defined roles and obligations. Part of the agency role is to take the initiative in facilitating cooperation and mutuality, and finding meaningful ways of involving families, in order to help meet the needs of the person with mental retardation.

The agency may offer the family support and educational programming around topics such as philosophies of support, or family roles in the lives of persons living out of the home. This may done as part of the admission process or other times. Topics related to death and dying may also be areas where the agency can support and educate families. These topics include the living will, funeral pre-planning, and decision-making around handling illness and death in the family.

Supporting secure relationship experiences is a basic part an agency plan to support grief care needs.

CHAPTER 6

Experience in a Grief Group

In a grief processing group for sheltered workshop participants after the death of a peer, I had a remarkable experience. Though others have suggested to me that I have read more into it than is really there, I say in response to this that I am reporting my experience, and that I believe the power and symbolic meaningfulness of the words spoken by group members is not my invention, though how it is described would certainly be different if someone else were there and telling the story about what happened. And, while in other cases in this book a sense of meaning developed through the inter-action of the client and the therapist, I was, in this situation, not actively interacting with the group, and was more a mere witness to the unfolding group experience.

I am obliged to recount this, and know that my subjective reaction says more about what happened than any attempt I might make to be merely objective. In any event I was astonished and awed by what was said in the group that day. My deep respect for the protagonists in this story, and their extraordinary empathic gifts, humbles me. I have, over the years, witnessed several incidents when a person with mental retardation has expressed him or herself with a sensitivity, clarity, simplicity, incisiveness, and immediacy that has stripped away the everydayness and debris that normally clutters my awareness, and struck me like a flash of lightning. What Emily shouted at the others in the grief group that day was very attuned to the grief dialogue occurring in the group, simple and direct, a masterful therapeutic intervention. But, also, her asking "the question" expressed her *own* experience of the question that she raised for the group, how intuitively and deeply she was in touch with both what the group was experiencing, and the question that she addressed to the group.

Here is the story. A workshop participant, Jacob, had died, and I was asked to facilitate a group meeting for his peers to talk about his death and their experiences of his death. Around the conference room's big table members took turns expressing their grief.

I'm upset.

It makes me feel sad. That's why I'm crying.

I miss him.

I'll miss him a lot. He was nice. I liked him.

He was my friend. He took a stroke. He was out with staff and wasn't feeling well.

While there was a sure and quiet sense of connection in the shared experience of the group members, there was also unexpressed sadness in the air. After a number of participants had talked about what happened when Jacob died, and how they felt, a silence fell over the group. It seemed to me that the group was sitting together, much more deeply together than at the start of the group. After sharing grief thoughts and feelings, the group seemed to feel comforted and bonded, each by his or her self-expression of grief in the group, and in their mutuality. In this bond there was, at that moment, also a more secure feeling of privacy, as each group member seemed to be sitting with his or her private self absorbed in self-reflection, and doing this together.

Then someone began to cry. I felt he was releasing a pain that was in the whole group—that the group had coalesced in the felt mutuality of the pain of each person, and he was expressing this while the rest of the group was silently in tune with him. The group continued to sit quietly with the crying person. After a brief time, raising his head, the man who had been crying noticed the person across the table from him, and, perhaps seeing a sad expression on the person's face, said,

I'm sorry I upset you. Sorry I cried.

Whether there was here a defensive and adaptive function of turning away from his own pain and experiencing it through and in concert with another, or whether it was guilt that generated and was expressed in this thought—it expressed, in a group dynamic way, an action in which the group members had bonded, an empathic, guilt-based identification among the members. His apology was an act of *taking care* of the man who was sitting face to face with him across the table. There was no overt quid pro quo, but it was the way the supportive mutuality of the group was carried and expressed by this individual. The mutual receptivity and the tender openness to grief feelings among members was unusually strong.

The words, "I'm sorry I upset you. Sorry I cried," evoked tears, or *gave permission* to the person to whom these words were addressed to cry, and he cried. For a long moment the group continued to sit in silence while this second man cried. Then, the whole group at once broke into tears, and verbally expressed sadness. Out of the chorus of weeping, one person said,

I want to leave now. I'm too upset to talk about it.

Another said,

All I can say is he gave us laughs sometimes. He was a wonderful person.

"I saw him on the stretcher," rejoined someone else; "I wanted to go with him."

Then it happened. Emily, the young woman sitting next to me jumped up and started waving her arms, pointing at the person who had just said that he wanted to go with him, and vehemently shouted,

How would you feel if you died! How would *you* feel if you died! How would *you* feel if you died! How would you *feel* if you died! How would *you feel* if you died! How would *you feel* if you died! *How would you feel if you died!!*

Everyone responded to her.

I'd be sad.

I'd be angry.

Angry. I'd be angry that I died.

I'd be scared.

Emily then said,

It's scary. Like a mystery.

And then she fell silent, again.

I was astonished at her outburst. Emily's speech was usually very poorly articulated and she spoke infrequently. She was so brutish in her social presentation of herself, that the sublime beauty, psychological sharpness, cognitive power, mastery, and boldness of her insistent questioning caught me, all the more, by surprise. Suddenly, I heard the question in my own soul: "How would you feel if you died?"

I was struck through and dumbfounded, while group members were simply recognizing the feelings of grief they had about the deceased, and experiencing and expressing feelings about their own mortality that were mostly similar to feelings about the death of their friend. The group members seemed calm, peaceful and very much in touch with themselves, their grief and each other. For the group it was comforting to reflect on their mortality together this way, but for me it more shocking than comforting, though I did, also affectively register the comfort the mutual caring, tenderness, safety, and healing among group members.

Emily had taken someone's saying, "I wanted to go with him," and heard in this a thought of her own dying. The man who said it no doubt meant leaving with the living Jacob who was sick, so that Jacob would not be alone; he was expressing a protective attachment and a feeling of missing Jacob. But Emily heard something different in these words. She heard "going with him" to mean *dying*. He was dead, and Emily imagined her own dying and articulated it as a question. Her comment on her own feelings, "scary and mysterious," was, coincidently or not, the same feeling I was struck by when she pounded home the words, "How would you feel if you died?" I felt an astonished and frightening awareness in me of my own death, and I took this to have been communicated to me and inspired in me by her speech. By *her speech* I mean the whole dramatic presentation, including the way she composed and expressed a frightening and mysterious awareness of mortality that she experienced as the thought of dying. Her expression was an act of intelligence, humanity, and courage that I had not expected to find in someone who seemed just a moment before to be not in any way in touch, let alone deeply in tune with, the psychological and spiritual significance of grief and death in the experience of others, and in her own self.

References Not Cited in Text on Mourning and Mental Retardation

Barbara, T. (1989). Training staff to care for dying clients. In M. C. Howell et al. (Eds.), *Serving the underserved: Caring for people who are both mentally ill and mentally retarded.* Boston: Exceptional Parents Press.

Barbara, T. V., Pitch, R. J., & Howell, M. C. (1986). *Death and dying: A guide for staff serving adults with mental retardation.* Boston: Exceptional Parents Press.

Ben-David, N., & Mansdorf, I. J. (1986). Operant and cognitive intervention to restore effective functioning following a death in a family. *Journal of Behavioral Therapy and Experimental Psychiatry, 17:3,* 193-196.

Beufus, J. A. (year not known). *Communication about loss and mourning. A curriculum of death education for the mentally retarded.* Byesville, OH: Guernsey County Board of MR/DD.

Bihm, E. M., & Elliot, L. S. (1982). Conceptions of death in mentally retarded persons. *The Journal of Psychology, III,* 205-210.

Borfitz-Mescon, J. (1988). *Parent-written care plans: Instructions for the respite setting.* Boston: Exceptional Parent Press.

Bogden, R., & Taylor S. J. (1989). Relationships with severely disabled people: The social construction of humanness. *Social Problems, 36:2,* 135-148.

Brasted, W. S., & Callahan, E. J. (1989). A behavioral analysis of the grief process. *Behavior Therapy, 5,* 529.

Carder, M. (1987). Journey into understanding mentally retarded peoples' experience around death. *Journal of Pastoral Care, 41:1,* 18-31.

Craft, M., Bicknell, J., & Hollins, S. (1985). *Mental handicap: A multi-disciplined approach.* London, England: Bailliere Tindall.

Crick, L. (1988). Facing grief. *Mental Handicap Nursing, 84:28,* 61-63.

Deutsch, H. (1984, December). Assisting mentally retarded individuals through the grief process. *Links*, pp. 12-13.

Deutsch, H. (1985). Grief counseling with the mentally retarded client. *Psychiatric Aspects of Mental Retardation Reviews, 4*:5, 17-20.

Eliott, D. (1995). Helping people with learning disabilities handle grief. *Nursing Times, 91*:43, 27-29.

Emerson, P. (1977). Covert grief reactions in mentally retarded clients. *Mental Retardation, 15*:6, 46-47.

Gaventa, W. (1988). On death and dying: A guide for staff serving developmentally disabled adults. *Mental Retardation, 25,* 387-388.

Griffiths, D. L., & Unger, D. G. (1994). Views about planning for the future among parents and siblings of adults with mental retardation. *Family Relations, 43,* 221-227.

Hedger, C. J., & Smith, M. J. D. (1993). Death education for older adults with developmental disabilities: A life cycle therapeutic recreation approach. *Activities, Adaptation & Aging, 18*:1, 29-36.

Heller, T., & Factor, A. (2002). Permanency planning for adults with mental retardation living with family caregivers. *American Journal of Mental Retardation, 96,* 163-176.

Howell, M. (1989). Grief counseling. In M. C. Howell et al. (Eds.), *Serving the underserved: Caring for people who are both mentally ill and mentally retarded* (pp. 327-379). Boston: Exceptional Parents Press.

James, I. A. (1995). Helping people with mental retardation cope with bereavement. *Mental Handicap, 23*:2, 74-78.

Kauffman, J. (1994). Mourning and mental retardation. *Death Studies, 18,* 257-271.

Kaufman, A. V., Adam, J. P., & Campbell, V. (1991). Permanency planning by older parents who care for adult children with mental retardation. *Mental Retardation, 29,* 293-300.

Kennedy, J. (1989). Bereavement and the person with a mental handicap. *Nursing Standard, 4*:6, 36-38.

Kloeppel, D., & Hollins, S. (1989). Double handicap: Mental retardation and death in the family. *Death Studies, 13,* 31-38.

Koocher, G. P. (1973). Childhood, death, and cognitive development. *Developmental Psychology, 9,* 369-374.

Lavin, C. (1989). Disenfranchised grief and the developmentally disabled. In K. Doka (Ed.), *Disenfranchised grief: Recognizing hidden sorrow* (pp. 229-237). Amityville, NY: Baywood.

Lipe-Goodson, P., & Goebel, B. L. (1983). Perception of age and death in mentally retarded adults. *Mental Retardation, 21*:2, 68-75.

Lutcherhand, C. (1998). *Mental retardation and grief following a death loss.* The Arc of the United States. www.thearc.org.

McDaniels, B. A. (1989). A group work experience with mentally retarded adults on the issues of death and dying. *Journal of Gerontological Social Work, 13*:3/4, 187-191.

McEnvoy, J. (1989). Investigating the concept of death in adults who are mentally retarded. *British Journal of Mental Subnormality, 35*:2, 115-121.

McLaughlin, I. J., & Bhate, M. S. (1987). A case of affective psychosis following bereavement in a mentally handicapped woman. *British Journal of Psychiatry, 151*, 552-554.

McLaughlin, I. J. (1996). Bereavement in the mentally retarded. *British Journal of Medicine, 36*, 256-260.

Moddia, B., & Chung, M. C. (1995). Grief reactions and learning disabilities. *Nursing Standard, 9*:33, 38-39.

Moise, L. E. (1985). In sickness and in death. *Mental Retardation, 16*, 397-389.

Mount, B., & Zwernik, K. (1989). *It's never too early. It's never too late. A booklet about personal futures planning.* Minnesota Governor's Planning Council on Developmental Disabilities.

Naragon, P. J. (1994). Death and bereavement: Issues for older adults with mental retardation. *University of Missouri-Kansas City Institute of Human Development: Fast Facts on Aging, 11*, 1-7.

Nelson, M. & Febeis, A. (1988). *Grief, death and dying.* Community Health Education Network of the Association of Retarded Citizens Minnesota.

O'Nian, R. (1993). Support in grief. *Nursing Times, 89*:50, 62-64.

Oswin, M. (1985). Bereavement. In M. Craft, J. Bicknell, & S. Hollins (Eds.), *Mental handicap.* London: Bailliere Tindall.

Oswin, M. (1989). Bereavement and mentally handicapped people. In T. Philpot (Ed.), *Last things: Social work with the dying and bereaved* (pp. 95-108). London: Community Care.

Patterson, S. L. (1978). The grief mode: applications within the school. *Social Work in Education, 1*:1, 64-75.

Peters, L. G. (1983). The role of dreams in the life of a mentally retarded individual. *Ethos, 11*:1/2, 49-65.

Ray, R. (1978). The mentally handicapped child's reaction to bereavement. *The Health Visitor, 51*, 333-334.

Reid, A. H. (1972). Psychosis in adult mental defectives: I. Manic depressive psychosis. *British Journal of Psychiatry, 120*, 205-212.

Rothberg, E. D. (1994). Bereavement interventions with vulnerable populations: A case report on group work with the developmentally disabled. *Social Work With Groups, 17*:3, 61-75.

Seltzer, G. B. (1989). A developmental approach to cognitive understanding of death and dying. In M. C. Howell (Ed.), *Serving the under served: Caring for people who are both old and mentally retarded.* Boston: Exceptional Parent Press.

Singh I., Jawed, S. H., & Wilson, S. (1988). Mania following bereavement in a mentally handicapped man. *British Journal of Psychiatry, 152*, 866-867.

Sternlicht, M. (1980). The concept of death in preoperational retarded children. *The Journal of Genetic Psychology, 137*, 157-164.

Turner, J. L., & Graffem, J. H. (1987). Deceased loved ones in the dreams of mentally retarded adults. *American Journal of Mental Deficiency*, *92*:3, 282-289.

Wadsworth, J. S., & Harper, D. C. (1991). Grief and bereavement in mental retardation: A need for a new understanding. *Death Studies, 15*, 281-292.

Wadsworth, J. S., & Wadsworth, D. C. (1993). Grief in adults with mental retardation: Preliminary findings. *Research in Developmental Disabilities, 14*, 313-330.

Wood, J., & Jackson, L. (2003). Future planning among parents and guardians of adults with developmental disabilities in a residential facility. *The NADD Bulletin, 6*:3, 53-56.

Yanok, J., & Beifus, J. A. (1993). Communicating about loss and mourning: Death education for individuals with mental retardation. *Mental Retardation, 31:3*, 144-147.

Index

Doka, Ken, 7
Down's syndrome, 71

Empathy, 3, 4, 10, 42, 62, 100, 106, 115-119
Experience of self, 7
Exposure anxiety, 85
Expressing grief, 2, 6, 42,

Facilitation, 2, 3, 6, 8, 9, 11, 15, 17, 19-22, 24, 28, 37, 38, 42, 49, 91-96, 106-109, 113-115, 118
Familiar environment, 2, 13, 15, 30, 31, 34, 55, 86, 90, 109-111, 114,
Family, x, 2, 9, 11, 13, 17,18, 21, 22, 26, 27, 29, 21, 32, 35-38, 46, 48, 52, 56-58, 65, 68, 69, 91, 94, 105, 107, 109, 112, 114
Funeral, 8, 27, 38, 56, 116

Grandiosity, 69
Grave, 28, 35, 36, 49
Grief behavior, 3, 7, 42, 43, 50, 54, 59, 63, 64, 97, 108
Grief counselor/therapist, vii, 1-2, 10, 25, 31, 36-38, 42, 54, 90
Guilt, 14, 23, 25, 27, 35, 57, 63, 78, 80, 82-84, 102, 110, 115-119

Hand biting, 82-83
Heaven, 47-48
Helplessness, 6, 13, 24, 44, 57, 64, 70, 73-74, 80-81, 112

Irreversibility, 17-18, 34

Klass, Dennis, 30

Language, 9-10, 16-19, 27-28, 42-44, 54, 59, 64-65, 72-87, 106
behavioral language, 9, 21, 41-42, 44
choreographic language, 44
grief language, 2, 16, 41-42, 44, 46, 50, 106
Learning from experience, 2
Legacy, 62, 94
Loss of self, 13
Lutcherhand and Murphy, 27

Magical thinking, 71
Memory, 27, 29-30, 33, 59, 61, 107
Memory book, 29, 33, 107
Mnemonic, 33, 35

Narcissistic grief, 5, 13, 14, 22-25, 36, 46, 47, 57, 61,65-69, 84-88, 106-107
Non-functionality, 17, 56
Normal grief, 10, 44, 54, 69
Normalization, 34

Persecutory anxieties, 84
Placement, 21, 30-32, 45, 68, 86, 96, 102, 109-112
Planning process, 32,
Policies, 89, 91-92, 98, 103, 104, 118
Preparation, x, 27, 29, 31, 34, 89, 94, 111,
Program development, 2, 10, 21, 34, 38, 89-95, 103, 105, 108

Rando, Therese, 14, 28
Recognition, vii, 2, 7-13, 15-16, 18, 24-28, 35, 36, 42, 46, 49, 60, 63, 70, 72, 77, 79, 87, 91, 96, 103, 105, 106, 111, 120

ABOUT THE AUTHOR

Jeffrey Kauffman is a Licensed Clinical Social Worker (Pennsylvania); Certified Addictions Specialist (in drug, alcohol, and sexual addiction; American Academy of Health Care Providers in the Addictive Disorders); Certified Thanatologist (National Certification Review Board of the Association for Death Education and Counseling); Board Certified Diplomate in Clinical Social Work (American Board of Examiners in Clinical Social Work); and Board Certified Expert in Traumatic Stress, Diplomate (American Academy of Experts in Traumatic Stress). He maintains an active private psychotherapy practice in suburban Philadelphia, specializing in grief and trauma, including treatment of persons with mental retardation.

He has taught at Bryn Mawr College Graduate School of Social Work and Social Research and at the Center for Social Work Education of Widener University, and has consulted with more than 25 mental retardation agencies in direct grief support services for staff and clients, training, and program development.

Kauffman is the editor of *Awareness of Mortality* (Baywood, 1995) and *Loss of the Assumptive World* (Brunner-Routledge, 2002). He is the author of many articles on death and dying.

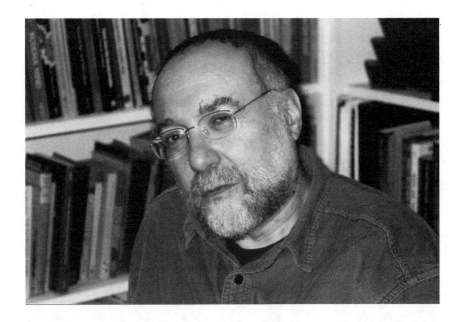